THE GENTLEMEN

YOUR STYLE BLUEPRINT

MTHOBISI MAGAGULA

cause or claims for loss or damages of any kind, including without limitation, indirect or consequential loss or damage arising out of use, inability to use, or about the reliability, accuracy or sufficiency of the information contained in this book.

For additional reading about men's fashion and style, visit https://mthobisi.fashion.blog/

Mthobisi Magagula is a 24 year old Writer based in Swaziland, Ezulwini and he is passionate about men's fashion, styles and blogging. This book *"**GUIDELINES AND TIPS FOR MEN TO WEARING IMPECCABLE OUTFITS**" is his first portable document book (PDF) for the year 2023.* Mthobisi wrote this book because of the enthusiasm he has for teaching men about dressing, how to dress, what to dress for events and most importantly he believes that a man can achieve anything he wants in life only if he dresses for it.

Mthobisi Magagula began his writing in 2020 at a time when the world was petrified about the devastating effects of COVID-19 which took a big turmoil and negative spin in many areas, industries, education systems and daily life as well. His blog "MENS FASHION & STYLE BY MTHOBISI" was incepted around May 2020 when the country was in lockdown, Mthobisi thought of creating his own digital platform blog where he would share his thoughts, ideas and solutions to men's fashion. He has been nominated for "BEST BLOGGER" two times since 2021 at the award ceremonies held in Eswatini such as the Swazi Fest Writers Awards whereby in 2022 he once scoped position 1 during the voting process in October last year.

He once made it to the top 10 of the Social Media Awards hosted by Swazi Boy TV entertainment in 2021.

Mthobisi Magagula going forward wants to impact as many men with his writing and also launch his own store and clothing brand one day as well as be Head of Marketing for a company are his long term career goals.

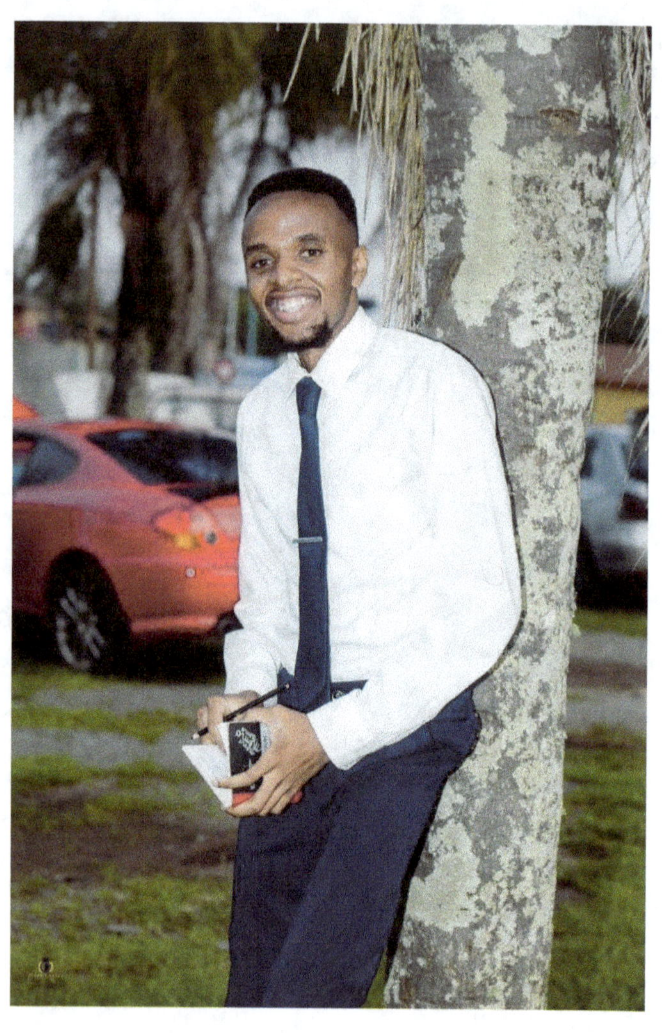

ESWATINI BASED AUTHOR AND MEN'S FASHION BLOGGER

MTHOBISI G MAGAGULA

CONTRIBUTORS

Meet our shining stars who
helped us throughout the
complete process!

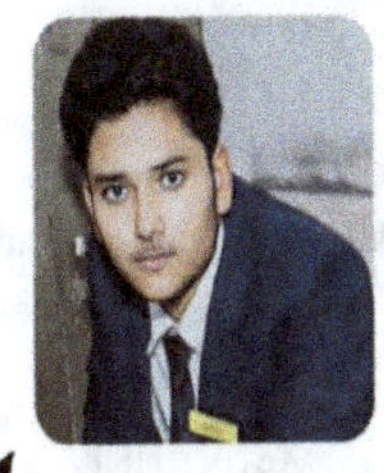

ANAS ANSARI

He is a talented artist with creative
mindset. His contribution has led to
remarkable designing of the book.
He is also an UPSC aspirant and
active team leader.

HEAD OF BOOK DESIGN

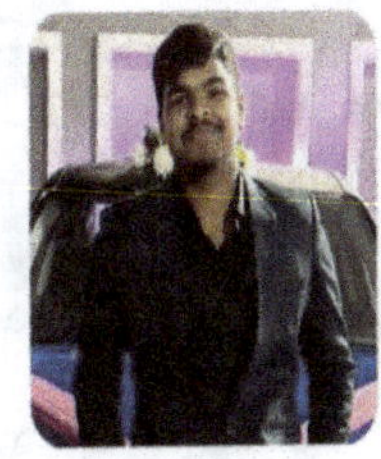

ARPIT BALA SAINI

He is the head of marketing team,
who contributed to the marketing &
promotions. He is also a content
creator and social media influencer.

HEAD OF MARKETING

CONTRIBUTORS

Meet our shining stars who helped us throughout the complete process!

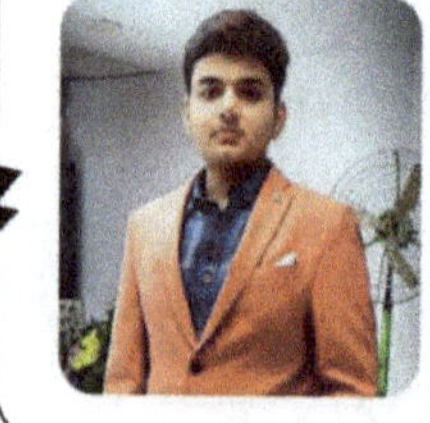

ALZAMA ANSARI

He is dedicated to promoting our team and making this book possible. His remarkable contribution speaks volumes.

MARKETING PARTNER

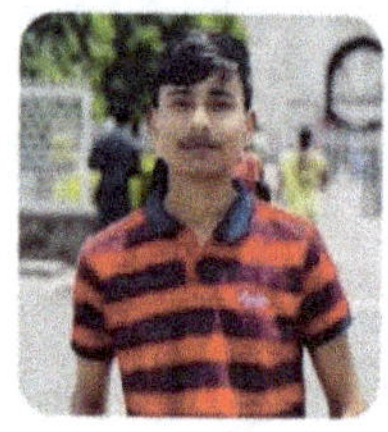

SAKSHAM GANGWAR

He's a social media influencer, helping us reach more people. With a vast network, he's a community champion, bridging connections with energy and engagement.

MARKETING PARTNER

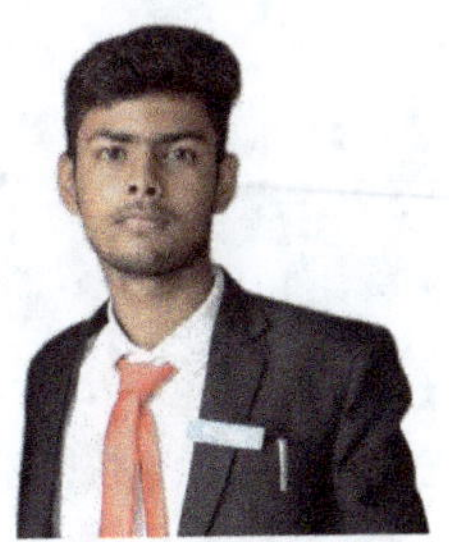

Mayank Gangwar
(Founder, Genius Words)

A book worth reading! In these pages, discover more than just style tips – unearth the art of self-expression, the confidence in every stitch, and the subtle language your wardrobe can speak. Redefine your style, step into your sartorial power, and make a statement that echoes beyond the fabric. Let this book be your compass to a wardrobe that speaks volumes without saying a word.

Dress well, live boldly!

Genius Words

An Initiative to Promote Aspiring Writers & Poets

 geniuswords1.wordpress.com

 contactgeniuswords@gmail.com

 @geniuswordsofficial

 @geniuswordsofficial

Table of contents

The practical sterling outcomes:

    A. Casual style evokes a feeling of relaxation

    B. Mixing the right casual pieces is comfy not sloppy

    C. Casual style grants you freedom to adopt your personal style

Part 3 – Tips for rocking accessories, casual style and fashionable pieces

Accessories men need to wear without breaking the bank

5 casual shirts men can pull off with plain suit colors

6 methods for dressing cordial everyday as a man

Dressing well as a man is for your betterment

How men can dress like they own the bank?

How to dress like a professional in the corporate field without suits?

How to dress sharp with white shorts in hot weather as a man?

How to dress stylishly as a man without trying too hard?

How to dress boldly in boots as a stylish man?

How to transform your life for the good as stylish man?

<u>**Introduction**</u>

Writing this is one of my goals this 2023 to exercise my writing craft given that I am a regular Blogger on a writing platform online called WordPress which is an application that enables an aspiring writer to pin down their thoughts in the form of a blog and one can even design a fully-fledged website there too. This book title is an idea that dawned in me this past couple of weeks around February and I said why not go for it and just speak my mind about it in the form of writing.

Studying men's fashion and style since I became a Blogger in 2020 is one reason why I wanted to write my own fashion book. This is not a hard book with science wrapped around it as if we studying rocket science but this is an idea that can be practiced in real life in regards to dressing sharp, men's tips for being stylish and lastly, this was written because of my aim and goal when I started a blog on WordPress and that was to help men dress better.

It really is that simple and if you are a man who wants to dress well and learn about the results you will experience when you are wearing your suit, blazer, boots, jeans and why nailing the fit of all these things gives you confidence, makes you to take radical changes in your life and even though this book will cover ONLY cold weather essentials and accessories in each of these six outfits doesn't mean you should stop there, you can apply what you have read here even during the summer season.

This book reflects my personality as well and my thoughts about the upcoming winter seasons which will be chilly and cold as weather predictors predict and why these outfits are a must have. So, I hope you will enjoy.

~Mthobisi Magagula

Don't let the cold spoil your confidence

As you dive deep into the contents and details of this book, there is one thing that must always be at the back of your mind and that is to always be confident in yourself and to let the fire burn even during the cold days when the cold and flu season has swayed by leaving the majority of men unconfident and having a low self-esteem to a point whereby they abandon dressing stellar as they should.

A quote by George R.R Martin that goes like this "Nothing burns like the cold" is a quote that means during winter or cold days the temperatures are harsh and penetrating like the burns of the sun in the exact same way that nothing burns like the sun during summer. Looking at how winter here in Africa is, it is evident that some parts of the continent are characterized by its wet and dry conditions due to the geographical locations. Editorial websites show that winter in Africa is generally warm and not as stiff as in other continents such as Asia and North America. Winter in this African continent is fairly mild to warm and it occurs between the months of June, July and August. However in other countries like Egypt winter starts from November up until April. From George's quote you can spot the way he is suggesting that people must possess confidence and keep the fire burning which can be applied to the contexts of men's fashion and style and how to style just six outfits during these upcoming winter months which will be cold, windy and wet in most areas.

<u>**The 6 Outfits**</u>

1. Business casual outfit plus cold weather accessories

The business casual outfit is one of the common dress codes for men and it is one that is not complex at all when styling one. This outfit just like the smart casual outfit is an outfit that comprises of button down shirts, sports jacket or blazers, dress boots, chino trousers or suit trousers, dress shirts with patterns and jeans.

One can even say this outfit is a relaxed style that cuts in the middle and sits in between dressy looks and casual looks. There are quite a number of blogs out there that can give you almost the same answer that business casual outfit is one that is less formal and one you can wear even at the office if you work indoors or at an event that needs you to dress a bit, the business casual comes to your rescue. Men are different and not all will usually go for the formal apparel, some are casual in nature, they grew up loving casual wear and in situations whereby they need to look their best, the business casual I bet is on top of their list.

The accessories in this outfit can be worn in different ways depending on the type of item you have on. If you are someone who loves sports jackets and blazers like myself, go for pocket squares, lapel pins and the tiny pins that can be seen closely like the one Presidents wear. If you are the guy who is not a blazer man but you want some type of jacket on, well my friend, wear a denim jacket, suede jacket with a dress shirt that has patterns and stripes such as the windowpane pattern and here you have the option of leaving the neckties at your flat and wear those dress shoes with chinos, if jeans are your pant combine them with Chelsea boots that are versatile in business attires be it business casual or professional.

Accessorize with headwear too, it is not just about the items you wear on the body but the head can be styled nicely and during those rainy and cold weather conditions you will not regret one of these accessories:

> **Scally cap**

Okay if you have watched Peaky Blinders in your lifetime then you probably know what a "Scally cap" is. One that you know since you can dress it on your head during cold days of course plus it really is not that expensive on shopping platforms like ebay. It can be defined in many ways, others call it a newsboy or flap cap.

This hat comes in a variety of patterns and colors which can also be beneficial if coloring is your mojo. The good thing about purchasing this hat other than it gives you heat on your head is that it can make you look taller since such hats give a man extra height. This hat as an accessory can be worn in the business casual dress code with a blazer, dress shirts with pattern and nice corduroy pants plus dress shoes or dressy boots. Hats in generally are stylish and they make the outfit unique.

➢ **Skull cap AKA the beanie**

Okay on to the next accessory in men's headwear and that is the beanie. This hat is obviously

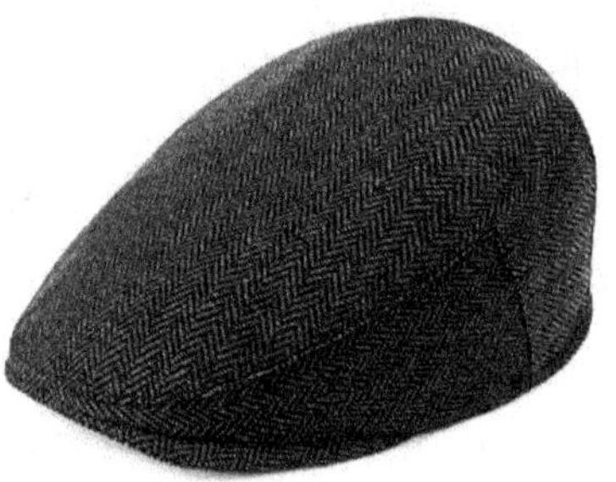

THE SCALLY CAP/NEWSBOY/ FLAP CAP

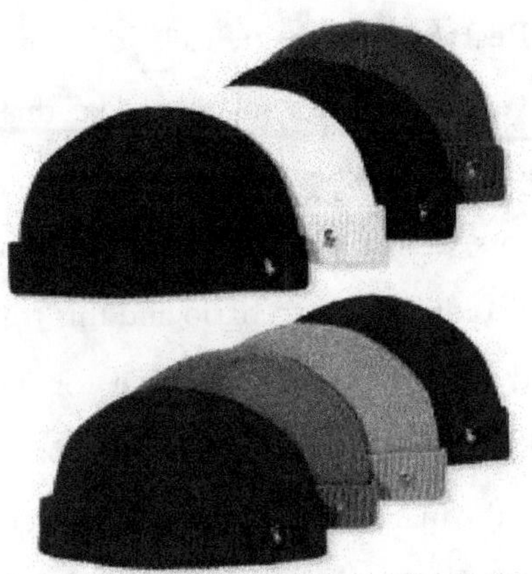

SKULL CAP/ THE BEANIE

2. Business formal outfit plus cold weather accessories

Okay on to the second outfit that keeps men safe from the cold days and that is the business formal dress code. This outfit is definitely formal and it needs your total commitment in styling formal wear like a boss. This is the outfit that is one hundred professional and worn by men who are of the working class and those in managerial positions such as CEOs, Managers, Shareholders, Head Teachers, Supervisors and those part of management like Head of department etc.. You get the picture.

Real Men Real Style website calls this outfit business professional and it is true, an outfit like this only needs formal apparel like neckties, a suit, dress shirts, dress shoes and black boots. Colors like black, red, blue, brown and grey are the go to colors in this scenario and this trifecta such as tie, shirt and formal trousers are ideal for looking like a professional. For the man who is not yet working, this style can be out of the man's league due to the expenses incurred here and most of these pieces are quite costly thus budgeting comes in handy to avoid risks such as debt. A suit in most occasions costs above one thousand to five thousand as the maximum payment needed for owning a well fitted suit.

Accessories needed in this outfit include:

- Scarf

- Leather gloves

- Overcoat

- Watch

- Tie bar

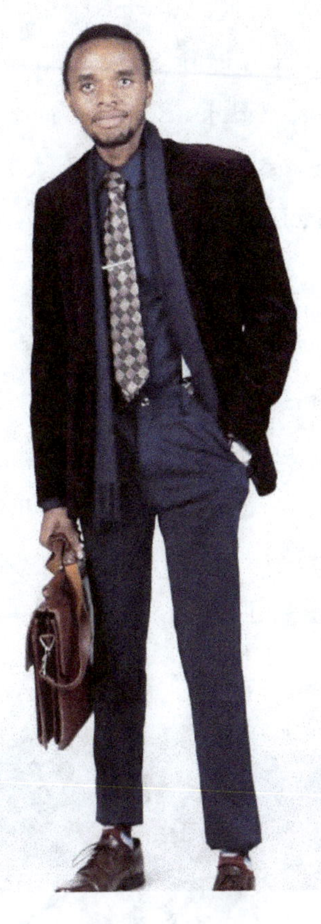

***BUSINESS FORMAL OUTFIT WITH A SCARF AS
AN ACCESSORY***

3. Classic 90s outfit plus cold weather accessories

Okay the third outfit that keeps men safe from the cold days is the classic 90s looks. These are looks that stand the test of time and will never be wiped out in the face of style. Looks like the ones icons Steve Mcqueen wore and those are turtlenecks, dad jeans, biker jackets, gloves, digital watches as accessories and bright colored windbreaker which were like rain coats or multi colored jackets.

For the colds I believe the wind breakers, leather gloves and turtlenecks will do some justice because they fight the cold and flu season right out of the door. There is a reason why stylish men who invest in classic pieces like these will never lose their confidence in dressing well it is because they invested in the 90s styles that were original, made from heavy materials and would always make a man look classic and clean.

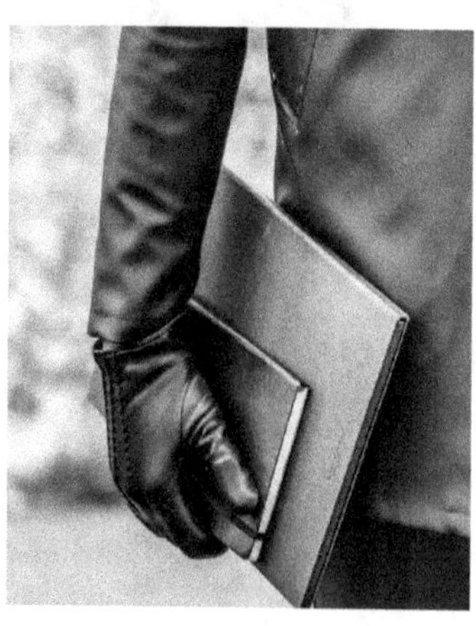

MENS LEATHER GLOVES ARE A CLASSIC PIECE

4. Smart casual outfit plus cold weather accessories

Okay the 4th outfit that keeps men safe from the cold days it is smart casual which is an attire that is geared towards casual wear but still needs to look a bit elegant and tidy. So, the men who have a love for casual wear do certainly wear such items in their day to day wardrobe.

This style requires a mixture of casual wear and classic wear. It is a fashionable look and it became a trend years ago and now the trending styles for 2023 are street wear chic where we see men pulling off chino pants with bucket hats and other cool pieces out there. Smart casual is the kind of outfit you can wear during casual events such as birthdays, soccer matches and a hangout with your buddies.

The accessories here can include bucket hats, tracksuits and bracelets and a scarf which is a non-negotiable accessory for beating the cold weather and for going out in public. If I were to take a guess what the majority of men wear on a daily basis it is smart casual outfits

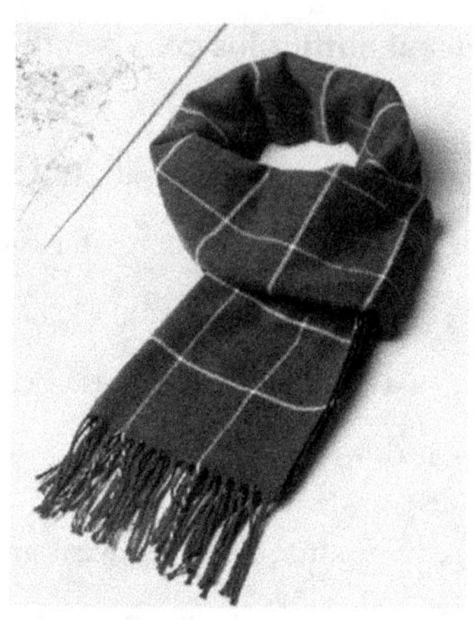

SCARFS ARE A NECESSITY IN SMART CASUAL

5. Black tie outfit plus cold weather accessories

This is a popular classic item in a man's wardrobe and it must include a blazer or a dinner jacket and for the tie a bow tie preferably in black so as to match the theme of 'BLACK TIE'. This outfit it is a tuxedo and the tux as it is usually called, first originated in America, USA to be specific and it was a menswear piece named after Tuxedo Park, a Hudson Valley enclave for New York's social elites and it first popped up in 1888.

The cold weather accessories here can be the leather gloves ONLY in my own experience as a Fashion Blogger because here less is more and only one or two details are mandatory. Also, an outfit like this is way more forma thus little to none details are needed. Just look at the example below

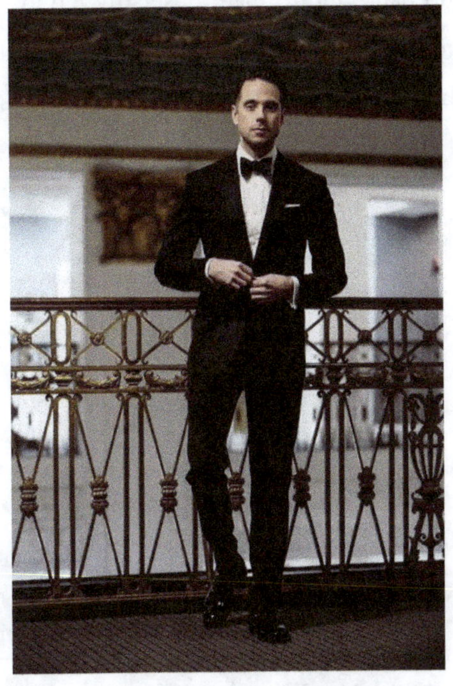

THIS IS BLACK TIE

6. Semi-formal outfit plus cold weather accessories

Okay the last outfit that keep men safe from the cold days it is semi-formal outfit. This one is like a business attire that requires no formal additions towards it like neckties, suspenders, bow ties and cufflinks or tie bars are not needed. Items like plain dress shirts worn collar less are ideal, chino pants and formal trousers tucked in with belts are required and for the accessories, a watch would suffice and if it happens to get cooler to cold, bring on scally cap or flap cap or a fedora hat to keep the head warm.

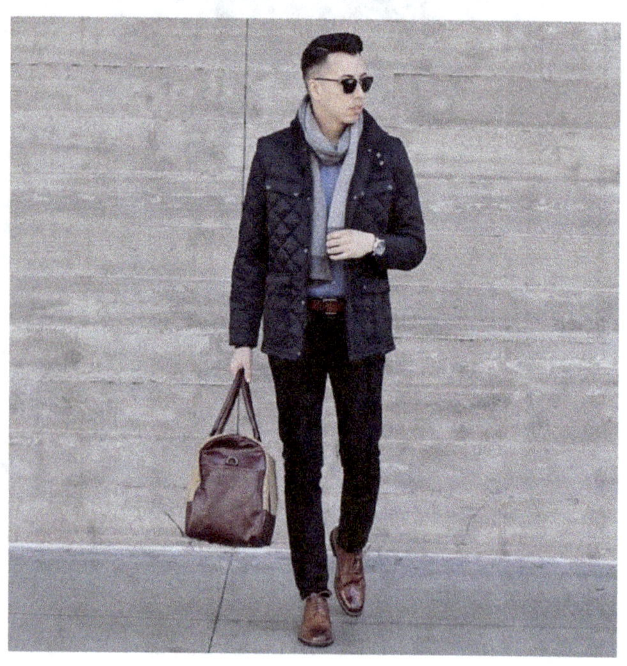

THIS IS SEMI FORMAL

Introduction to casual menswear

Casual wear is all around us, everywhere you turn to and everywhere your eyes land you spot several casual styles from both men and women. This book is an in depth analysis of the casual styles that men wear, why wearing fitted pieces is essential, the sterling outcomes of wearing fitted casual wear and what casual wear is not as well as the reasons why trends in casual wear are not for the older and matured man.

Casual wear in simple terms means wearing what feels comfortable and it is the simpler way of dressing light and cool. When thinking about casual wear the majority would say: Jeans, T-shirts, Sleeveless shirts, Shorts, Accessories, sneakers and chic colors such as bright yellow, greens, reds, purple, orange and more. On the surface that is true but the best way to dress pertinent in casual menswear it is not to appear too casual or in other words overdoing it as you dress casually.

This list comprises of items men need for casual wear to look radiant on their bodies and for their personal style:

- Fitted T-shirts

- Graphic t-shirts

- Plain shorts

- Flannel shirts

- Polo shirts both plain and patterned

- Headwear: beanies, caps & bucket hats

- Fitted jeans

- Loafers, boat shoes or summer shoes

- Chino trousers, accessories, sports jacket and casual blazers

The origins of casual style

Casual style in the men's arena dates back to the years clothing were manufactured and although we can't really say the exact year and day because the internet was still extinct and not existing back then but blogs online pin down what they believe is casual wear and from the look of the images these were clothing the men of that generation wore or should I say what the forefathers and ancestors wore. A reliable blog called Vintage Dancer which can be accessed online via https://vintagedancer.com inform us that the casual styles of the 1940s to 1960s was where casual wear took its inception and till date these casual pieces can be worn during the vintage shows and fashionable events that have a theme that says 'Vintage wear".

Vintage refers to ancient items that were there for years and still look original in the current century. Items such as vintage cars, watches, hats, schools and so on have a distinct and a never ageing appearance to them. The same goes for men's fashion and style, there are vintage pieces that are casual that never fade but are eternal in holding its motive which is to last forever.

Polo shirts, dress slacks, dad jeans and all other casual items were the ones that were worn and these casual items were fitted to the tee (Probably there was a tailor back then) and the amazing thing about casual wear it is that it is a sophisticated, comfy and relaxed style that is ideal for every day wear.

Vintage casual men as you will see from the pictures below wore polo shirts that were usually designed with prints such as the windowpane pattern and stripes, trousers that were dressed tight up a notch to the stomach area and as you spot the man from the right holding golf tool.

<u>1940s to 1960s Vintage casual wear for men</u>

These images below were extracted from the Vintage Dancer website – https://vintagedancer.com

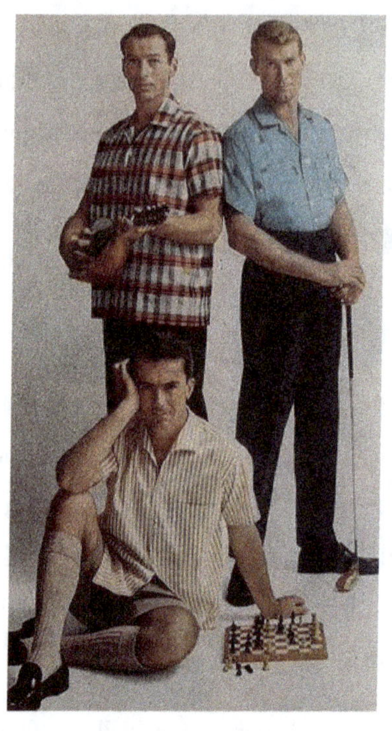

Looking at the casual wear of today, you can definitely spot the differences since now we have a bunch of casual items, brands and lots of designs that are suited for both young and old men. Skinny jeans, ripped jeans, oversized hoodies, casual prints, cross body bags, oversized shoes, sunglasses and necklaces that are glittering are the current casual fashion out there in the market.

1940s Casual Men's Style VS 2023s Casual Men's Style

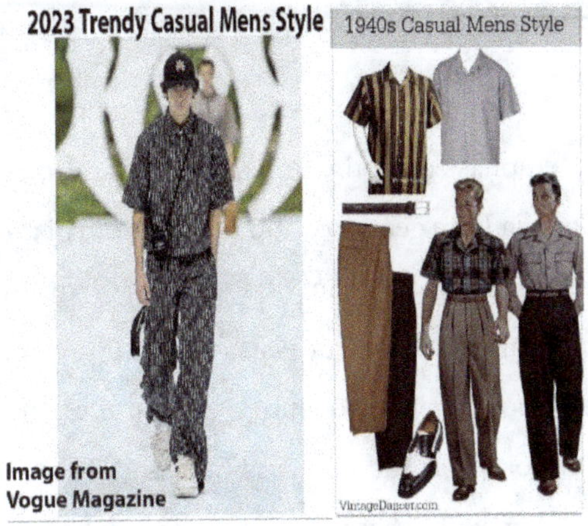

Why nailing the fit of your casual wear makes a man trustworthy?

Don't get me wrong, this heading is not at all implying that wearing casual wear makes you honest as a person or man but from a fashion and style point of view, the fit is the key aspect here that makes you seem as trustworthy to others.

Fit is very vital in nailing an outfit and it is not about the price tag here but the fit which means make sure you wear what your body size is looking for. I suggest reading some helpful information from this website called "Real Men Real Style" https://www.realmenrealstyle.com it has tons of information but the essential one you will grasp it is about fit. Fit is king and it don't matter what type of store you go to if what you purchase is oversized you have wasted a lot of money which would have been used for other things.

Seriously, as a man who writes about men's fashion and style, I emphasize on the urgency of fit and these days of social media I can get to pick up images from platforms such as Pinterest and Instagram and although I may not touch the garment physically but just by looking I can see if that jacket is too tight for a chubby guy or too big for the little guy. Proportion is the takeaway here and if your body size doesn't align with what you put on, leave it because it won't do you justice in dressing the part.

The fit makes you trustworthy because you look neat and like a man who has all his affairs in tip top form and order. Nailing the fit is like cooking, if you cook with the right ingredients in the table you are guaranteed to cook up a storm compared to making a dish you have never made before, using wrong ingredients and sauces leading to the meal looking sour and it will probably taste like that to a guest instead of the meal looking scrumptious.

Fit goes hand in hand with function and then the fabric too. See the fit here is like a pyramid, for the pyramid to balance, all these three items here: fit, function and fabric can be mixed and shifted but they all say the same thing and that is "This is how you look the part".

If the pyramid were to fall it means then these three steps that always aid men to dress better have not been implemented for a successful execution. It is like placing a big piece on top of a small one, the outcome there is "Downfall" because there is no balance.

Function

The function goes hand in hand with the fit, fit being the top because it is the smallest icon and you can see how the balance works. The function part refers to occasions, events and ceremonies that need a man to dress the part depending on the type of event of course.

For casual wear, the ideal ceremony for rocking chic casual pieces it is the social gatherings, leisure and informal events such as birthdays, friend's farewell, attending concert, exhibition and fairs. Okay, I know for a fact that people vary and there are those who would wear casual even on formal settings and events, it is just how life is and it is unpredicted that's for sure.

A man wearing a suit in a casual setting well, others won't notice and won't even care but for a man who cares about his appearance and wants to explore casual wear, my take is drop the suit when attending informal gatherings because the suit was designed for essentials work tasks such as an office setting, weddings, formal functions and more.

NOW ON TO FABRIC!

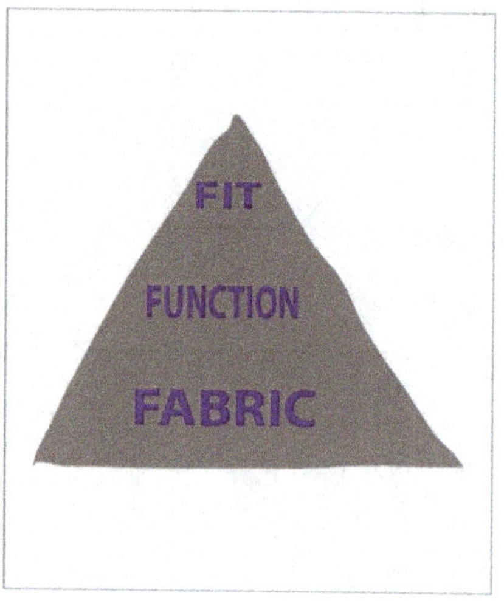

The style pyramid every stylish man needs to know

Fabric

Okay for fabric, I am not going to dive deep into explaining the fabrics out there but these illustrations below should make your mind understand why fabric is needed and why the right fabric makes you look reliable.

a.   **Linen Viscose blend fabric**

According   to   Pinterest (https://alohafabricsexport.com/), this linen viscose fabric is a natural linen with viscose fibres and the material is excellent leading to a durable fabric ideal for any occasion. From my view as the Mens Fashion Blogger, this fabric is super fresh and breathable that is perfect for casual wear, imagine the t-shirts, shorts, flannel shirts, polo shirts all coming from this material, it is amazing when the final product comes out and just by looking without touching you can see that this cloth is made from the best materials and linen viscose is one of them.

b. Cotton fabric

The second fabric that is ideal for casual wear it is the cotton. As usual cotton is soft on the skin and for summer time even winter wearing cotton on your outfits signals a well sharped outfit and you always look great. Fabrics goes hand in hand with both fit and function. This fabric is ideal too because it is very breathable and my favorite of all numerous fabrics out there. Hey I am not a fashion designer but I know which fabric is right and which one is itchy and not right.

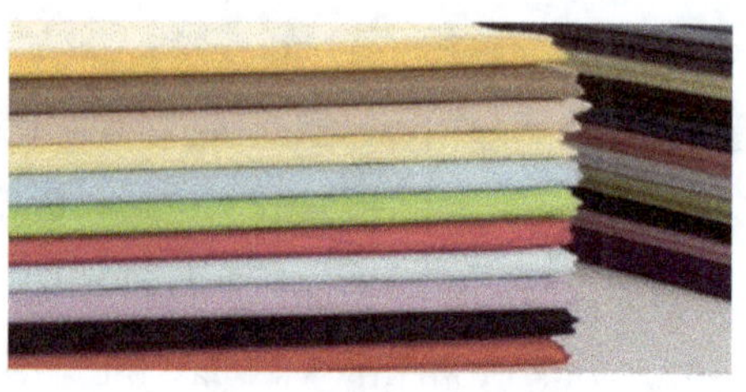

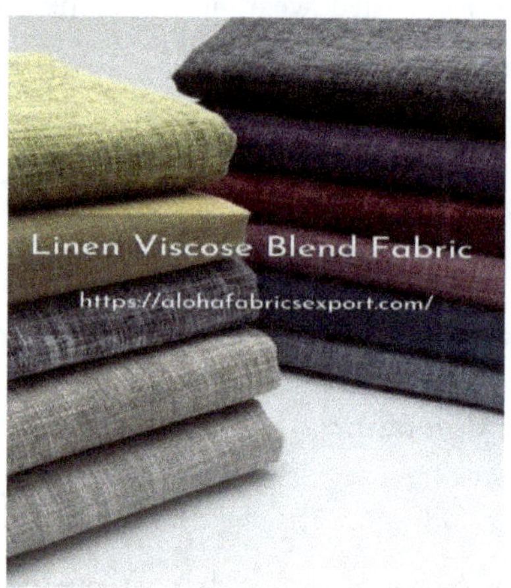

This is the Linen Viscose fabric ideal for casual menswear

Following trends is not for the mature man

Can you imagine a man aged 50 pulling off ripped jeans, cross body bags, street style and the latest trendy clothing that has a youthful attitude? It looks irregular and insane because we expect a man with that age to dress appropriate, to dress for this age and to wear presentable clothing. I mean who wants to look 20 when they are already 50, when the time has passed by these older geysers should just look back with pride and not try to change the time that has evaded way too much to dress like a street style kid.

Hey, I am not saying it is not possible for the older men to look young but they need to wear the right casual pieces such as polo shirts, linen shirts, white sneakers and boots even but not chest out floral shirts, tattoos on their body and trying to look like a Justin Bieber in that outfit, it will never suit his age group.

Just look at this picture below, it is not for the mature man whose about to go into retirement.

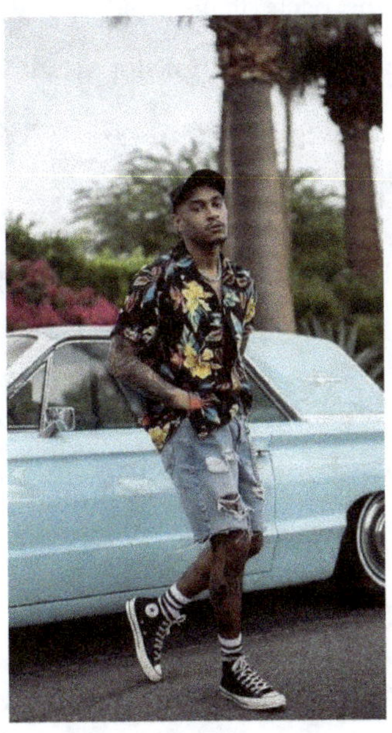

PART 2

A. Casual style evokes a feeling of relaxation

Onto the sterling outcomes which is the main purpose of this PDF book and that is wearing fitted casual pieces leads to a feeling of relaxation.

Imagine it is a scorching hot day, on a Friday morning, you have been invited to attend an event , say a party at your friend's place, you want to come dazzling in style but you don't want to be overdressed yet you want to look the part and be relaxed at the same time. Well, for the man with this issue toppling the back of his head, this is what he must wear, something relaxing yet not sloppy but suitable for that party. Say, the theme is smart casual wear or ultra-casual, here are the items a man needs:

- Polo shirt/T-shirt with prints not logos
- Plain shorts
- White sneakers/Loafers
- Bag(cross body bag or others) for accessory
- Watch
- Sunglasses for the sun/Cap

IMAGES OF HOW TO WEAR ITEMS THAT EVOKE A FEELING OF RELAXATION LISTED BELOW:

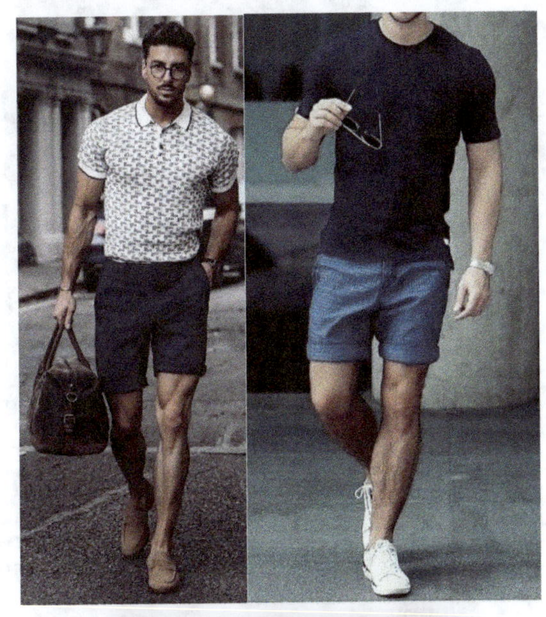

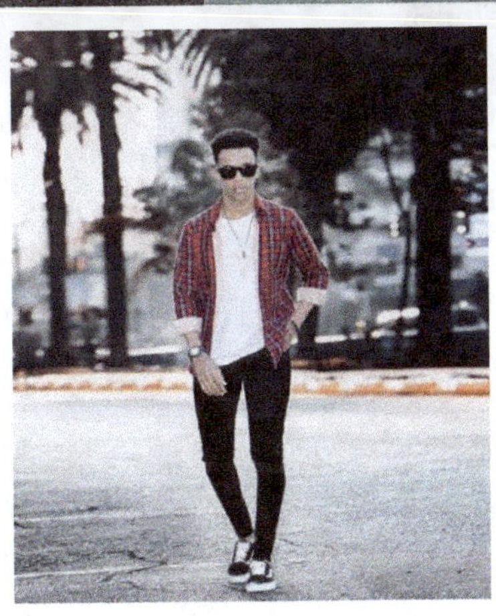

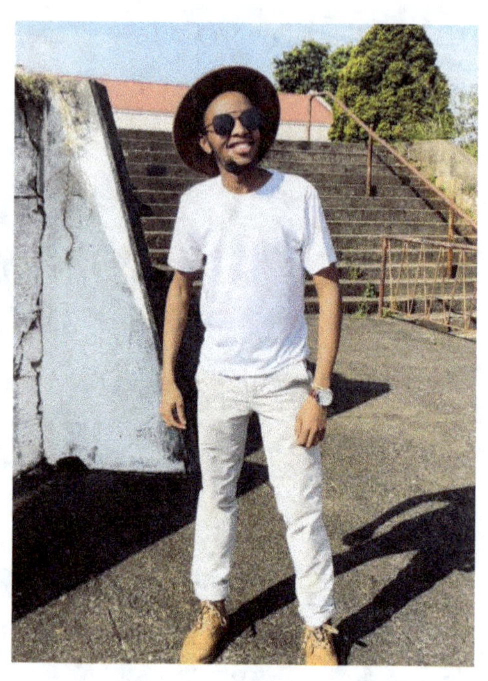

B. Mixing the right casual pieces is comfy not sloppy

Okay here the outcome of mixing the right textures, colors and items leads to a comfortable style and not sloppy. What makes casual wear sloppy is the fact that you trousers are falling, you wearing wrong color combinations and you refuse to wear a belt. Well, the images below will give a man ideas on how to start dressing like this when wearing casual wear and not forgetting the fit.

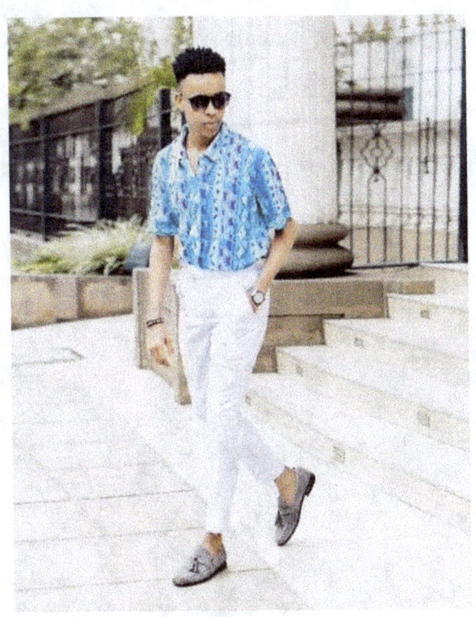

A mix of blue and white is always a winner if you want to look cool and chic in casual. Try this color combination, master the fit and you will win.

C. Casual style grants you the freedom to adopt your own personal style

Everyone has his style and he ensures that he wears it again and again because it has become a part of his life. Now, to adopt your personal style, master the fit, as you have read above the style pyramid, fit is king. A t-shirt, jeans, polo shirts and sneakers are all key components of a well put together casual style. The best way to adopt your personal style it is to explore the casual wear until you find what truly resonates with you and which style speaks to you the most.

The below images are examples of casual outfits men need to try to give their personal style a leg up:

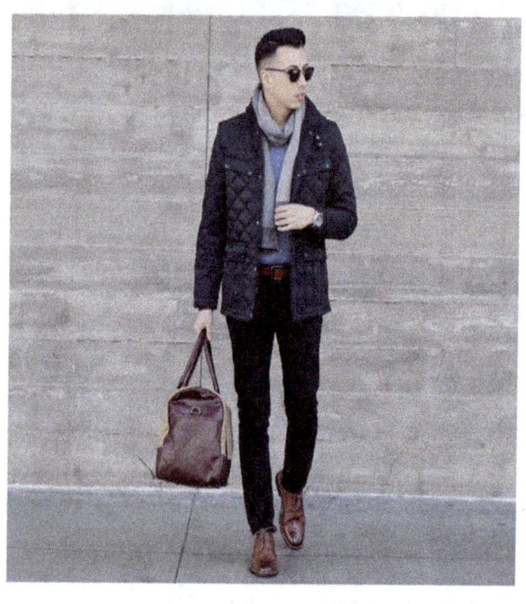

FOR THE CLASSY MEN WHO WANT TO LOOK SHARP YET CASUAL

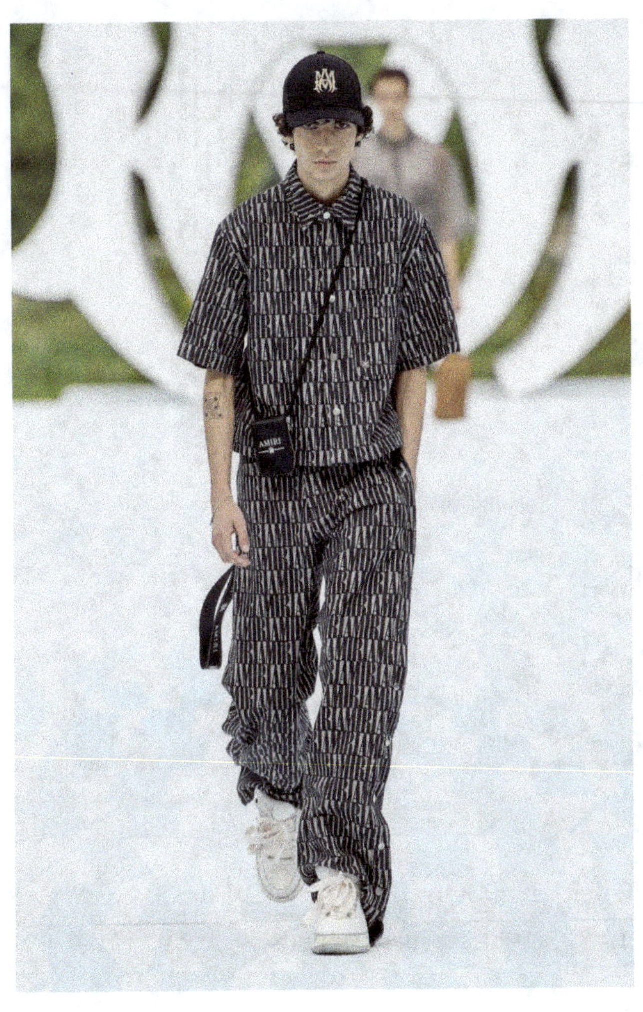

FOR THE MEN INTO TRENDS (YOUNG PEOPLE)

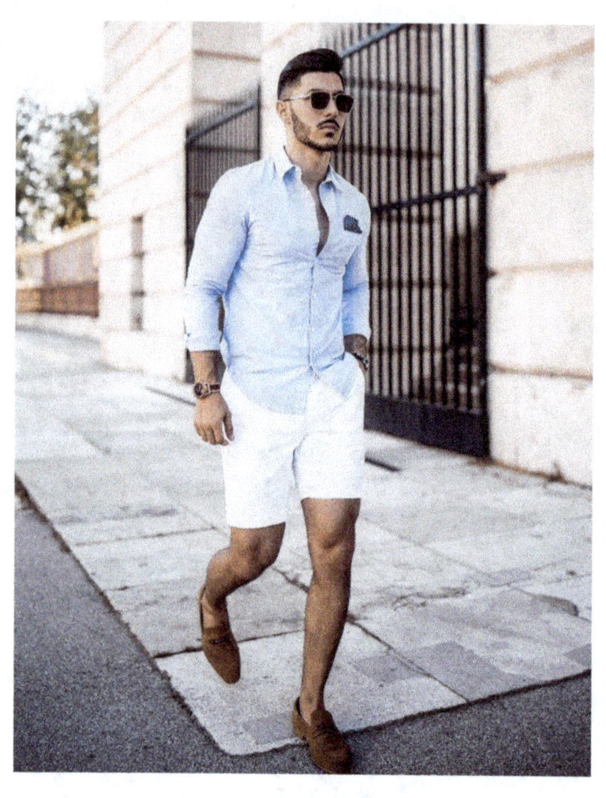

FOR THE COOL GUY WHO WANTS TO WEAR DRESS SHIRTS WITH SHORTS

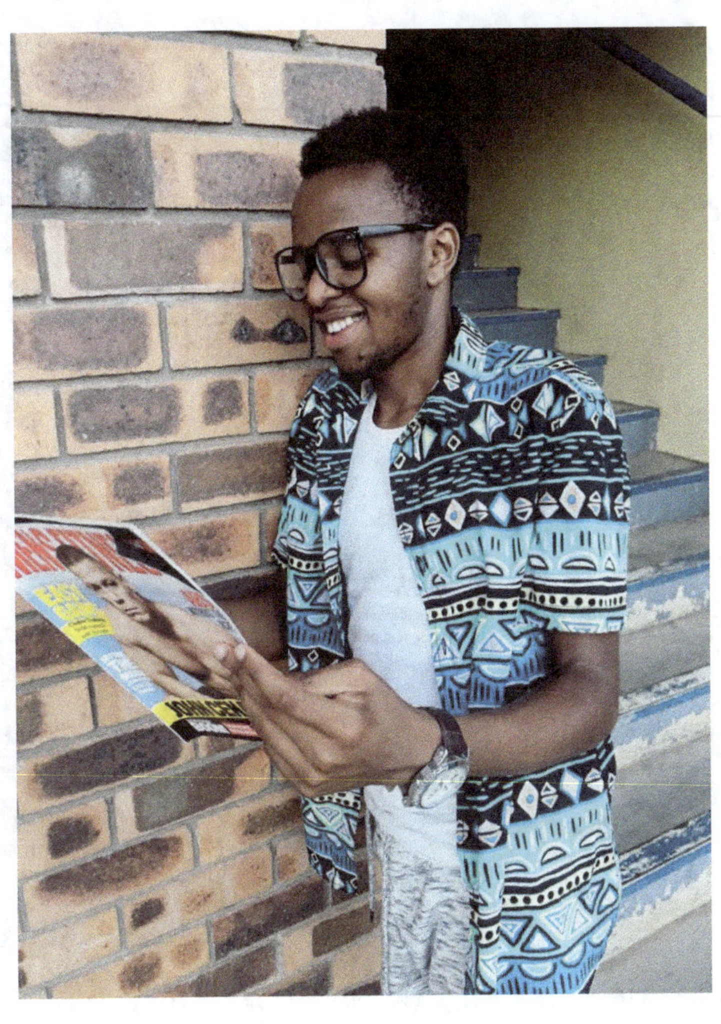

FOR THE MEN WHO WANTS TO DRESS CREATIVELY IN CASUAL

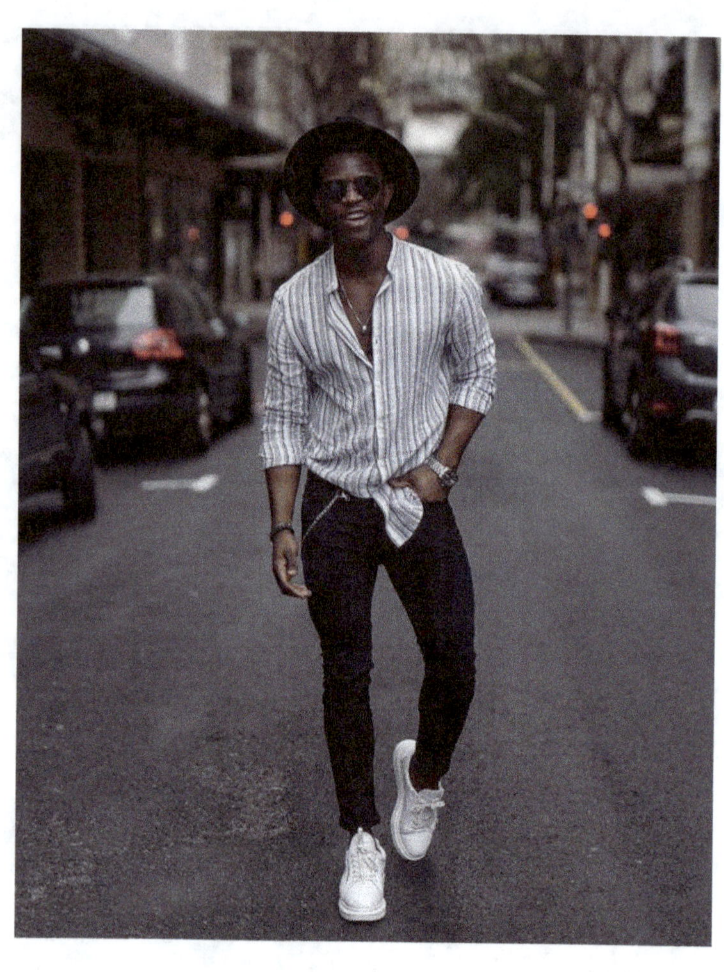

FOR THE MEN WHO WANT TO ROCK STREET STYLE YET IN A PRESENTABLE MANNER

ACCESSORIES MEN NEED TO WEAR WITHOUT BREAKING THE BANK

It really is not that expensive to own a couple of accessories in your wardrobe as a man with fashion and style sense. Accessories are like spices you add in your food to ensure that the meal not only tastes palatable but also ensures that the meal looks appealing even to a guest who would love to give a bite of it. There are literally a vast majority of accessories out there in the market and so many options are available to men ranging from formal wear accessories such as bow ties, watches and cufflinks to casual wear accessories such as Panama hats, watches, sunglasses, t-shirts and boots. This blog will distribute the need of owning five accessories especially in your casual wear and those are: Panama hats, T-shirts, Watch, Sunglasses and a pair of boots.

1. Panama hats

In 2021 I published a blog post about "Hats can upgrade your style" and I wrote about the types of hats we have such as: Ascot hat, Newsboy, Flap Cap and Beanies but for the purpose of this blog, I will do an in depth analysis on the Panama Hats. Panama hats have been around for centuries and are just an elegant plus timeless fashion piece men wore and the start of the 20th century has seen such hats gain popularity and have been worn by many prominent figures such as Presidents, Actors, Celebrities and even a regular man who want to dress without breaking the bank can buy a Panama hat. The reason why this hat is a need is because it allows ease and the hat is a breathable material which is perfect to be worn during hot days or the summer and spring season. According to a source from Google, Panama hats are the seaside and tropical accessories men would wear at the beach hence they are to be worn during extremely hot days.

2. T-shirts

T-shirts can be defined as a casual light item that is usually made from cotton and this is a very soft fabric. T-shirts date back to the 19th century when American laborers cut their jumpsuits to cope with the summer heat. The first T-shirt was invented during the Spanish American War in 1898 and was used as an undergarment. Nowadays, T-shirts are not only used as an undergarment but as an accessory you can dress it up alone even with a panama hat and a nice blazer to look classy and elegant. For casual wear scenarios owning a T-shirt is the best thing a man can do and buying a white t-shirt is ideal because it is a versatile piece to own.

3. Watch

Okay as a man of style I can tell you that owning or let alone buying a watch is a lifesaver. It is not just an accessory but it is like a relationship with time, when you have a watch on you are never late in most situations because the clock is there to guide you and if you work in an environment like teaching, a watch saves you from being late for teaching lessons and even students now that the academic year has started need to have a watch. Watches date back to the 16th to 17th century and the first watch was made by a clockmaker from Nuremberg called Peter Henlein.

4. Sunglasses

Switching to the upper body part of the face, the eyes which need to be protected from the sun rays thus the need of having sunglasses on. Sunglasses come in a variety of sizes, shapes and colors. According to www.pinkvilla.com, there are many sunglasses for men such as: Aviator sunglasses, Clubmaster sunglasses, Round sunglasses and Wayfare sunglasses and many more. For casual wear, sunglasses are an obvious accessory even if you are not a man of style.

5. Boots

Shoes are an essential part of an outfit. In fact, footwear is very key in every outfit you wear and the boots in my fashion opinion are a perfect shoe a man can ever own. I mean just look at the many benefits it carries with it such as: it makes a man look taller, it enables you to work with ease, it is comfortable and it is ideal for rainy days and it will never let you down in terms of scoring points on an outing with your friends or dates.

<u>5 CASUAL SHIRTS MEN CAN PULL OFF WITH PLAIN SUIT COLORS</u>

Suits are defined as a jacket and trouser made from the same fabric and there are incredible ways of styling a suit formally and casually depending on your preferred style and taste. Men don't need to wear a suit with tie all the time but they can absorb other casual pieces in their wardrobe such as casual shirts which are ideal for plain suit colors such as navy blue, grey, brown, white and red which is also known as burgundy. This blog post aims to address five ways men can pull off a plain suit with five casual shirts available in their closet and without further ado, let's hop in.

1.   **Navy blue, grey, brown, white and red suits can be worn with a casual polo shirt**

First shirt on the list of five casual shirts it is the polo shirt. The history of polo shirts date back to the 90s but that's for another day, a polo shirt is casual because it's design is casual looking at the sleeves, the buttons on the front are usually two to three compared to a long sleeve dress shirt with lots of buttons. With the polo shirt, it also needs to be well pressed like the dress shirt, meaning it needs to be ironed and I suggest men opt for solid plain colors such as brown, white, blue, black and red because they will match well with the suit. Imagine a blue suit with a white polo shirt and nice loafers, the outcome is a dashing elegant style. Also, polo shirts can be tucked in just like dress shirts so they are a must have if you want to substitute a white dress shirt for it and wear this look when going to a casual event such as a Friday party or brunch with your buddies.

2. Navy blue, grey, white, brown and red suits can be worn with a floral shirt

Okay the second way to dress elegant with a plain suit color is to bring in a floral shirt. This is a shirt that has floral and patterns in it, like the beach shirts men wear when they go to the beach. By the way, last year, I wrote a blog post titled "THE CREATIVE METHOD OF WEARING A FLORAL SHIRT AND BEACH SHIRT WITH A SUIT", is an informative blog post you will peruse. The floral shirt got its' name from the designers who designed pastel shirts such as the ones Indians wear and it is a very casual shirt. The sizes vary since we have short sleeve and long sleeve floral shirts.

Out of all these five suits, you are guaranteed to look dapper and elegant in this floral shirt and you can select any color you want on the shirt , imagine a brown suit with a pink floral shirt, it just looks exquisite. At the end of the day, it is up to the man to decide which suit color he wants to wear but I suggest the man play around these plain colors such as: red, brown, white, navy blue and grey.

3. Navy blue, brown, blue, white and grey suits can be worn with a solid T-shirt

The third item on the list is none other than the famous T-shirt which is the default casual shirt for the majority of men. The t-shirt is super versatile and that's why men wear it almost every day. In terms of dressing elegant with a suit, men need to bring in solid plain colors because those graphic T-shirts actually make your outfit look trendy or fashionable which is not a bad thing but for dressing sharp, plain t-shirts are the ones to use. Imagine this scenario, you have a presentation to deliver in front of lots of people like a public speaking challenge and you will be up there standing on the podium, you want to wear a suit but you don't want the suit and tie style, well, t-shirts are there as a substitution. A white, black, grey and blue t-shirt in plain colors is the best way to style your suit. I have pulled this look off countless times, so can you.

4. Navy blue, brown, white, grey and red suits can be worn with a collar less shirt

The fourth item on the list is the collar less shirt. Well, this shirt isn't worn often lately but it is there, some call the shirt with no collars a Chinese shirt and indeed this shirt has no collars only buttons that are going down. I used to wear this shirt a long time ago and it was a long sleeve but I believe a man can pull it off with a plain suit. They usually say there is a first time for everything so I too agree that the only way to be sure of your style it is to try it on. A white suit with a grey or red collar less shirt is perfect. Also, I suggest men follow "COLLAR LESS & CO" on Instagram to see what amazing shirts this brand or company has for men.

5. Navy blue, white, brown, red and grey suits can be worn with a flannel shirt

Did the thought of wearing a suit with a flannel shirt ever cross your mind? Well I suggest that you start thinking about it because wearing a suit with a flannel shirt is an awesome look. For the flannel shirts, go for those blue ones, white ones and black mixed with other patterns since the flannel shirt just like a flannel has textures and patterns like stripes of brown, white or blue. I happen to own one flannel shirt in my wardrobe and I have worn my navy blue suit with my blue flannel shirt and loafers or slip on covered boat shoes and the outcome was a sharp smart casual style. A suit can also be worn in smart casual situations by having one casual item which is the flannel shirt and it has to be tucked in, a tie is a non no here because the shirt is casual, so with the collars it is like a button down, it needs to not be fastened but let loose and some men even wear casual shirts like these showing off their chest.

Therefore, attempt to wear a plain suit with these casual shirts and you are sure going to look the part.

<u>6 METHODS FOR DRESSING CORDIAL EVERYDAY AS A MAN</u>

Dressing cordial is actually dressing nice. Cambridge Dictionary and Oxford Dictionaries define the word cordial as friendly, warm but polite as well as formal. When it comes to a man looking great, he needs to practice wearing nice pieces so that dressing cordially for him becomes a walk in the park. This blog post will point out six methods that are guaranteed to assist a man to dress cordial leading to the process being a no brainer.

1. Wear a watch

An article by fashion beans which can be accessed via this link – https://fashionbeans.com/article/how-to-dress-well-men/, gives one solutions about the need of wearing a watch. A watch is like a piece of art, it says a lot about a person and the best way to acquire one it is to go for the right size that will fit your wrist and you need to be practical whilst buying one. The watch should be an accessory a man can wear in almost all his dress codes such as black tie, business formal, cocktail attire and ultra-casual. I believe that of all the accessories that are gracious and look great on the eye, a watch is a must have plus it guides you so that you become punctual.

2. Grooming is a key skillful tactic in dressing nice

Recently, I wrote a blog post titled "6 Ways to dress like a high level achiever" and grooming was one of those ways. Grooming is about self-care in particular the skin that needs to be maintained by bathing, cutting your finger nails, looking after your hair and shave the head and beard(optional) if it is too long. This is super practical and easy because it ensures you look nice. Truly taking care of yourself as a stylish man yields many returns because for one you get welcomed everywhere you go.

3. Invest in dark colored boots

I like boots one is that they give me extra height as a man and secondly, they are very warm plus versatile especially when styling clothes during winter or cold days. Chelsea boots for instance are a must have especially the darker colors like black because it is a proper color for looking nice and it will match even a nice suit on a cold day. Also, dark boots can be dressed down with jeans, crew neck sweater and leather jackets, suede jackets or any casual jacket you own.

4. Mix and match your accessories

Okay this is for adding fashion sense to your closet and that is don't be shy but be super confident when styling your clothes. Firstly, when wearing formal wear, wear not just the watch but mix it with a bracelet, necklace and rings because it shows that you are not afraid of being flamboyant, interesting and cool. However, this rule here is a bit tricky because if you don't tone it down with your accessories you will overdo it. Thus, two to three accessories are all that's needed not five to ten.

5. Apply good smelling perfumes

I have talked about fragrances and wrote countless blogs about the need of spraying perfumes. By the way, do read my old blog post "Looking good should be accompanied with pleasant perfumes" and your eyes will be wide open about how to apply perfumes and when to apply them so that you not only dress nice daily but you smell nice daily too.

6. Plan the day before which outfit you will wear

This one is very significant because if you want to always shine and look proper, select an outfit the night before because it saves you time plus it shows that you are putting the effort in looking the part. Yes, you won't dress well daily since some work in environments that are different thus suits won't be a daily bread for them but try to iron and pick the outfit yesterday.

DRESSING WELL IS FOR YOUR BETTERMENT AS A MAN

In as much as life is meant to be enjoyable, dressing well is also meant for your betterment as a man so that you gain confidence, dress for success, ensure people trust your word and above all for your betterment so that your life makes meaning and the best way to live life to the fullest it is by dressing well.

Here are the benefits of dressing well as a man:

1. Men who dress well are not second guessed by people in terms of their profession

Imagine you wake up every day and you go to work, say you are a Doctor and when you enter the work station, people give you that look and their facial expression gets irritated, now what is the cause of this? It is because you didn't dress like a Doctor, you look like you slept in the cemetery. Say you are a well-known doctor yet you entered the hospital wearing shorts and you didn't even shower maybe you were running late, that appearance doesn't do you anything justice at all because people will be disappointed with what you have worn at work, I mean wearing shorts as an honored doctor is completely unprofessional. Thus, dress like a Doctor, wear that doctor's coat like the other doctors, shower and apply colognes or a perfume to smell nice and people will not even think twice that you are Doctor.

2. Men who dress well receive tons of respect

This is a fact that men who adorn themselves accordingly by dressing well do receive vast amounts of respect and that respect makes them grounded and the man ends up respecting others as well in the process. For instance, you want to make a turnaround in your life and you no longer want people to mock you be it at work, school, your home or the community you reside in. Start by dressing well and don't end there , surround yourself with other men who are going places in life, who respect themselves and doing so will affect your life heavily.

3. Men who dress well are the best and are seen as game changers

Just like the game of football, there are players who are known to convert the game from being stalemate to being a winner. To be seen as a game changer and to be considered the best in whatever you do, dress well in your nice clothing, be it a suit, business casual attire and even smart casual wear. These dress codes will always make you like a game changer who has his eye on the ball. Even the best coaches in football like Pep Guardiola of Manchester City dress well when going out to the pitch to coach and monitor his players so that they win the game.

Therefore, as you read this information here I am fairly certain that you will do better as a man and dressing well is done for yourself to be better and not for the other person.

HOW MEN CAN DRESS LIKE THEY OWN A BANK?

There is a quote that is a norm in the fashion industry and it says 'Dress like you own a bank not like you need a loan from it", and it is true. Dressing in that order of being someone who is a millionaire is a great feeling because your dress code signals a person who is rich and that is why men need to dress that way. Dressing in a way that seems like you are rich is a great example because it gives a man confidence and it makes the man to be engrossed at the task at hand plus he feels like he is holding all the assets in his hand. This blog will give out examples of outfits men need to wear so that their appearance looks like that of a Bank Owner even if they are not into banking.

1. **Wearing a well fitted suit allows a man to look like he owns a bank**

Well everyone knows that a well fitted suit is a great example of how to project an image of being wealthy. Even women that are in the corporate world wear suits when going to work because it defines their reputation and it makes them look professional. I have written a blog post about "5 Must Have Items For Men To Dress Professionally" and that blog is somehow similar to this one in terms of dressing like a professional and a well fitted suit be it a 3 piece suit or a two piece suit grants a man access to looking like money bags. Truthfully, men who work as Investment Bankers, Auditors, Accountants and Chief Executive Officers in the banking industry wear suits almost each week since it is their profession.

Now you don't have to work in banking to wear a suit. You can save money and once the funds are available head over to the best menswear store and purchase a suit that fits your body size and you will be grateful for doing so since the suit slims your silhouette and makes you look like the man in charge. Add details such as pocket squares on the suit and a watch to dress stylishly and elegant you will certainly appear like those guys who work in corporations.

2. Get a quality formal shoe such as brogues

I have written a blog about shoes in February that men need to fall in love with and dress shoes also known as formal shoes were amongst the list. Okay you all know that men who are into the corporate world wear classy shoes like brogues so it will be easy as taking a candy from a baby when styling your shoes that will make you dress like you own the whole bank. Shoes like black oxfords or brown brogues are ideal because they can be dressed with suits, with jeans too and they are very comfortable. We all know that banks deal with financial services and the staff there dresses formally in most occasions so can men who want to project an image of "Authority" dress like that. Quality shoes like these can be dressed with suits as usual and even dressed casually with jeans. However, the disadvantage here is that shoes like these are expensive thus a man needs to work hard to buy them.

3.   Always wear a belt with your formal ensembles

Belts are a must have because they give your appearance a neat feel to it and you look presentable as well as respectable. I also wrote a blog post before about 'How to dress simple yet presentable?' and a belt was among the items discussed on that blog. Belts are super affordable, from less than 200 bucks you can get a quality belt that you can wear at work, when delivering presentations or at important events such as birthdays and graduations. Belts can be dressed with suits, jeans and even shorts such as linen shorts. Men who work as Bank Managers always wear a belt because they want to not only be seen as rich but they want to dress respectable so that people get to appreciate their work ethics.

4. Have a professional bag such as a briefcase to look like you packed millions in that bag

Men who work at banks always or sometimes bring briefcases to work because they are incredible for packing important documents or work items that they will need at work such as files and papers. In my view, briefcases are ideal and wonderful bags for looking sharp, for storing work files and for keeping confidential information inside without allowing others to open it easily. Briefcases are great for doing business if you are a Manager. Such bags look great with suits and are typically worn by Lawyers, Doctors, Bankers and anyone who wants to store important documentation or gadgets inside. Trust me, investing in a briefcase is a lifesaver and you do look like you possess lots of millions on your name.

So, as you can see it really is not that hard to dress like you own a bank as a man and here is the trick, you need to shop for quality over quantity.

HOW MEN CLOTHED IN SUITS BECOME BETTER THAN COUCH POTATOES?

Suits are my favorite outfit selection in my closet and I have been in admiration with suits since before I was a Men's Fashion Blogger. Suits are defined as a jacket and trouser made from the same fabric and there are many detrimental improvements and advantages of wearing suits hence men who are clothed with suits are seen as proactive, energetic and powerful based on appearances. This blog will describe the benefits of wearing suits at work, during prominent events and whenever they feel like looking sharp.

1. **Suits were designed for functionality and they make a man look proactive**

There is a quote that says "A suit is the uniform of success and elegance" and in one way or the other that quote is evidence that suits carry with them this sparkle of success and elegance no matter your age, background or social ethnicity. Suits need to be well tailored that is the trick and they are very functional in terms of fit, comfort and being proactive whilst wearing it. Men in suits (yes you can't state the personality of a man firsthand) appear proactive, that is, they know what they want in life and they don't mind dressing for it.

2. Suits come in many vents thus they make a man look well mannered

Ever notice that couch potatoes are those guys who don't want to lift a finger to help, they are always demanding plus they lack in manners, they talk anyhow as if the world is theirs. I am not at all suggesting men in suits are perfect since they are those dressing like a sheep in a wolf's clothing but from first perceptions a man in a suit is expected to be well mannered who uses forms of addresses such as MR. OR MRS. When talking to people. Most men in suits wear suits with different vents such as the single vent and double vent.

3. Coach potatoes procrastinate yet men in suits don't mind starting from ground zero

Yes this is another reason why men in suits are far better than men who just linger around the house or sit at the coach with no plan to make themselves better in life. A suits man is always able to focus at the task and doesn't lay off or postpone their goals in life. Honestly, I would believe a man wearing a suit that he has changed his life around and he is venturing into business tenders with the motive of making a profit to sustain himself. Even if the man has no money or capital to take off but by just wearing a suit, people get to trust that man because of a wonderful exhibit of first impressions. Also, if a man is planning to get a loan to start a business he is highly likely to get it from the bank because he is dressed like the shareholders or employers of the bank.

4. Confidence level shoots up when wearing a suit than a coach potato sitting alone in the corner

According to www.realmenrealstyle.com , men wearing their best get to adopt high levels of self -confidence because the man feels good. Suits are not uncomfortable but they are unfamiliar in this case. The first time I wore my suit when I was graduating from University, I was very confident and driven with this positive outlook I had in life and I was happy with my accomplishment. It always feel good to dress to the nines when accumulating your achievement be it a loan, certificate, new car, new house, new job, new dog or pet(optional) and any other accomplishment you would love to get from this one life you have. Compared to a coach potato or lazy bones who rely on others for survival just like this CHATGPT that will create a line of lazy people because it does all things for you within minutes or even seconds especially in writing blog posts.

Therefore, I urge men to avoid being lazy and to always dress the part specifically suits that were designed for that, to help men look good for their special day.

HOW TO DRESS LIKE A PROFESSIONAL AS A MAN IN THE CORPORATE FIELD WITHOUT SUITS?

The corporate field is quite a complex one for all people for both men and women included. This field requires determination, team work, mental acuity and education to be able to climb the corporate ladder as they usually say it. A corporation can be defined as a group of people who come together to create a single entity. In legal terms, this is a company or organization that was created for people to pull goals together with the aim of making a purposeful profit. Now, to dress like a professional just like those accredited Bankers, Investors, Lawyers, CEOs, CFOs, Legal Advisor, Marketing Manager and all those other pro titles in the corporate world, needs a man to invest in professional looking pieces such as dress shirts, neckties, jeans, boots, v-neck sweaters, watches, glasses and other acute outfit pieces that are suitable for this field.

1. **Invest in black as a color for one or two of your sharp outfits**

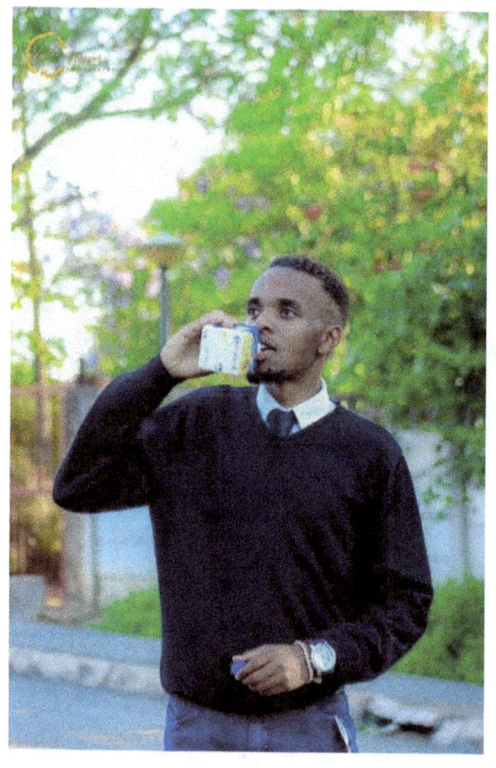

Black is one of the formal colors and for good reasons, it is classy and a quiet yet powerful color. In other countries, they only wear black when attending funerals and other mourning activities whilst for some white is worn for funerals, it depends on which country you reside in. In terms of the corporate world, to reach that stage of being a legit professional, a man must invest in his education and also his wardrobe. Black is one of the easiest colors to find in the market, a black v-neck sweater is ideal for corporate wear without always putting on a suit. Why? It is because the color itself is appropriate for work wear and also the sweater can be paired with a white dress shirts underneath (see featured image of this blog post) and even a necktie in black too. This is such a clean look and for the trousers, you don't have to wear a formal one unless the management of that corporation or agency doesn't permit its staff to wear other casual trousers but jeans are okay for this semi-formal look and they must be well fitted and with no rips like the ripped jeans. For the shoes, go for dress shoes since these are fine for office wear but also try boots like Chelsea boots in brown or blue or black colors (they are perfect for professional appearance) looks good with this semi-formal outfit. The detail here to look like a pro is have one or two items of your outfit with the color black.

2. **Instead of the suit, wear a white dress shirt without the tie with plain suspenders and formal trousers (for hot weather conditions)**

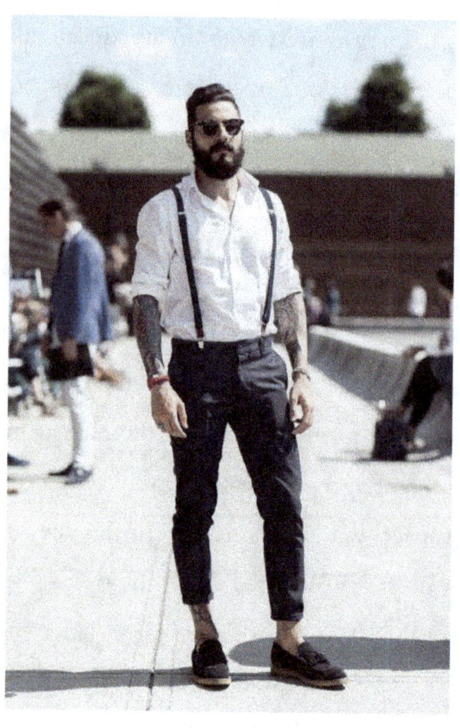

This is another way to add some style to your corporate wear and that is instead of wearing a full suit with a tie, do wear a white dress shirt with the plain suspenders such as navy blue, red or black instead of the belt and you can show off your formal wear with those braces or suspenders of yours and this outfit is ideal for hot weather conditions whereby a suit or a blazer is not required but you still want to dress like a professional.

It depends on the type of corporations you work for because some provide their staff with a dress code they must abide by and wear all the times when they go to work. However, some agencies don't have a dress code and as a former employee for an advertising agency, there really wasn't any dress codes there, guys wore their clothing but you can step up your work wear with such outfit pieces such as suspenders, watches and shades but keep it simple.

3. Tuck in your shirts

Corporate men wear suits as usual and these are the Lwayers, CFOs, Managers, Supervisors and even the Interns, they dress sharp and neat. It is just how the corporate world is, everyone there represents the company so they must look proper for incoming clients and business investors who happen to pass by. This is to say, the men need to tuck in their shirts, a Manager doesn't need to wear a suit but he can tuck in his shirts to look like a professional. Before people can say you are a pro first dress the part, it is the little things such as the tucking in, ironing the clothes and taking care of the skin. I recommend men check out John Henric on Instagram and on social media platforms to see amazing men's items like shirts and accessories that are great for corporate wear and at affordable prices.

Visit http://www.johnhenric.com/ to see the latest men's style and fashion.

HOW TO DRESS SHARP WITH WHITE SHORTS IN HOT WEATHER AS A MAN?

Hot weather happens now and again and it is the best weather condition for most males because they get to wear their favorite casual outfits. It is during summer seasons whereby hot weather brims out often and there are a variety of ways to dress sharp and fierce when the weather becomes extremely sunny or hot. Out of all the trousers out there, men's shorts are preferably the best ones to reveal to the world and mixing them with other sharp pieces in your wardrobe to look good because the weather permits of course and the best shorts are made from linen and cotton since they allow air to flow and are breathable. This blog post will list examples of ways men can dress sharp with white shorts when the temperature reaches its maximum degrees. (By the way, dressing sharp needs a dress shirt, blazer, polo shirts, loafers and a belt since they can all be worn formally with a suit too)

- **Matching white on white is a great way to look clean and pure yet sharp**

  Ever seen an all-white outfit displayed on stores or better yet worn by people you see on the way. Matching white all the way from the head to the toe is a great way to look sharp and bonus science tells us that lighter colors reflect on the sun and they bring out vibrancy and radiance on the outfit and they deflect on the sun rays so that you feel relaxed and not overheated. For instance, wearing a white dress shirt with white shorts and white sneakers and adding a bit of accessories like a watch leads to a vibrant style. If you are ever in doubt about matching colors that will make you look sharp, wear all-white or all black and you will see yourself looking exquisite.

- **Wear a blazer and white t-shirt to pull off a business style that is relaxed**

  Okay I know most men don't usually wear blazers with shorts but in my view they can look sharp with this outfit combination, they just need to try it on. I have tried this outfit on as you can see below and it looks so neat and sharp. This is the outfit you can wear when going to the boardroom on the weekends because it is relaxed yet well combined with the blazers and to add style, throw in the pocket square on the blazer to look elegant. For the shoes, go for sneakers since they are ideal or low top loafers.

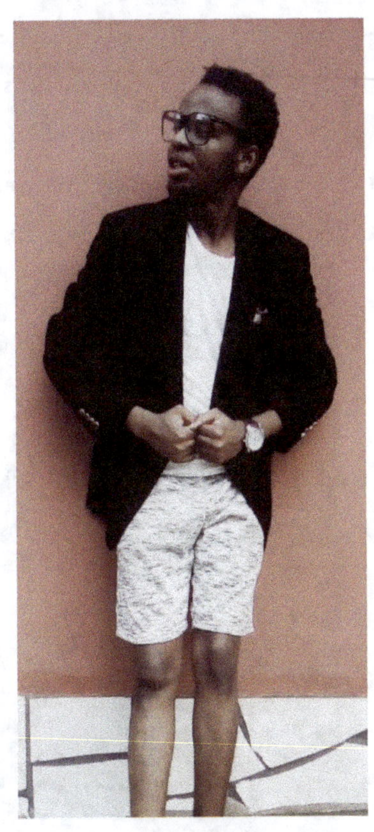

- **Wear shirts such as dress shirts in dark colors or go for polo shirts with loafers**

From my experience the best color combination it is black and white and here a navy blue or black dress shirt with white shorts and loafers is an awesome look to pull off and as you can see below these guys pulling off this look which is ideal for hot weather and summer time. If long sleeve dress shirts are not your bread and butter, don't sweat it, there are short sleeve polo shirts you can use to your advantage to look elegant in the process. For footwear, loafers are ideal or if you don't own one, go for plain white or black sneakers or low tops.

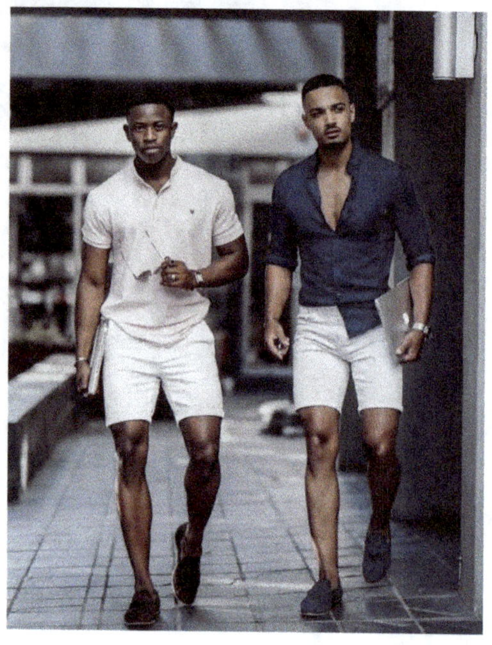

To conclude, with all these three options available to you, you are guaranteed to look sharp during hot weather conditions.

HOW TO DRESS STYLISHLY AS A MAN WITHOUT TRYING TOO HARD?

Dressing stylishly is actually a walk in the park for the man who has mastered the art of dressing well daily. In fact you don't need to spend thousands and thousands in money to purchase outfits that will make you look very stylish and elegant. This blog will dish out ways to dress with style as a man without stressing yourself out. So, read on closely gents and don't just end here reading, apply these techniques in your personal wardrobe and you will surely stand out with your style.

1. **Invest in basic staples such as solid T-shirts which can be worn with high classic pieces**

Okay so you get the idea, investing in solid colors such as blue, white, grey and black in a T-shirt actually creates a versatile look. I have written a blog post in the past about "***Ways to infuse a T-shirt with style***" and this post describes the need of basic solid staples in a T-shirt because they can be easily matched with all the items in your wardrobe even high classic pieces such as suits, fedora hats, overcoats and even a cane which you wear when wearing a three piece suit. Also, I suggest colors that are mostly dark and for the lighter one white and grey are ideal since they can be interchangeable with other pieces even the shoes such as sneakers and boots as well as trousers like jeans.

Lastly, solid colors in T-shirts are quite affordable on the market for less than 50 bucks you can come out with a quality T-shirt which you can infuse with a suit, suede jacket, denim jacket, jeans and good looking shoes like boots or sneakers. Say, you are attending a gala event but you don't want to wear the dress shirt with your nice suit, you can opt for a solid T-shirt especially black or white since these are more formal colors.

2. **Add fun accessories like a watch , sunglasses and bracelets without breaking your bank balance**

I know there are men who want to dress in high end brands and wear expensive accessories but not all have that privilege since people aren't the same. So, the best accessories that will still make you stylish without trying to dress like a celebrity it is to just buy a watch, sunglasses for those sunny days and a bracelet to add spice and variety to your style. Stores such as Mr. Price, Woolworths and Edgars to name a few can grant you such accessories that won't hurt your pockets in the process.

3. Invest in a hat which you can wear casually and formally

This is another way to dress stylishly as a man without trying too hard and that is to invest in hats. In 2021, I wrote a blog about *"Hats can upgrade your style"* and the content I dispatched there will open your eyes to see the need of owning a hat which is also versatile for casual wear and formal wear occasions. Thus, hats such as Fedora hats, newsboy and those classic panama hats are just perfect and I own two pairs and they just add so much style to my outfit even if I decided to wear casual that day. Of course, weather predictions will always vary daily but if the weather permits grab your headwear item and go rock the day with style.

4. Cleaning, exfoliating and applying fragrances to the skin is also considered being stylish

This is the easiest ways to appear stylish without trying too hard and that is to just take care of your skin, clean it or bath as they usually say, exfoliate the skin by applying skin products which I believe need you to invest your money so that you look fresh and rejuvenated. Also, let us not forget fragrances such as perfumes and there are a plethora of them in the market out there, buy one that evokes good emotions and make you feel comfy and at ease. Honestly, the best way to dress stylishly after putting on the amazing outfit it is to apply a perfume on the body and the outfit, people will notice and smell that fragrance which can give you tons of compliments. The best perfumes can give others assumptions that you are wealthy and you bath using those expensive skin products for men. So, you can see the power of grooming and wearing simple yet stylish pieces as explained above.

HOW TO DRESS UP BOLDLY IN BOOTS AS A STLYISH MAN?

Boots are like daily bread in the style arena and to show some style as a man, needs you to invest in a nice pair of boots. Boots generally are footwear you wear when the weather gets chilly to cold. These are shoes that are for work purposes and boots like the gumboots are worn when attending to the fields or ploughing fruits and vegetables in the yard. The style boots on the other hand, are different from the gumboots because they are designed for dressier situations. There are many boots out there at stores ranging from combat boots, duck boots, suede boots and the common Chelsea boots. This blog post will explain the innumerable ways men can dress boldly in stellar style with just one pair of boots.

1. **Black boots are a great choice for formal dress codes**

Okay, this is clear as day that black is a color that symbolizes class and aggressiveness thus it is the most formal colors in the market. A black suit worn by a man means business and most wear such a color when attending funerals and other important functions that needs you to look serious and solemn at the same time.

To dress boldly as a lion needs a man to buy black boots, preferably the Chelsea boot because it is classic and it does a better job of dressing you up especially during the cold weather seasons that have fallen upon us lately(My country Eswatini to say). These boots with formal dress codes such as black tie, business formal and even semi-formal to even casual looks sharp on the man.

If you admire formal wear such as myself, you wouldn't mind purchasing another pair of Chelsea's. This boot with a nice black suit and bow tie, looks very neat. The advantage of boots it is that it increases your height and they protect your ankles from tragic events such as falling.

The same goes for other dress codes such as business formal and semi-formal that needs a man to look his very best and dignified as if he was attending a significant event such as a funeral and wedding or graduation.

2.   Casual boots are a great choice for casual wear dress codes

On the other hand, there are casual boots that are an incredible staple for casual style. These boots include: the combat boot, derby boots, duck boots and dessert boots as well as suede ones. These boots are ideal for casual wear because they match well like twins with the other casual pieces in a man's closet.

A dessert boot in medium brown and also the colors play a big role in shaping a man's style to whether it is casual or on the formal side. A sports jacket with dark jeans and such dessert boot is a great way to dress bold casually. The best thing about sports jackets it is that they can be dressed up casually hence the dress code here is business casual that aims to strike a balance between formal and casual.

Sports jackets in grey, blue, brown, white, green, red and black even with little patterns with a t-shirt, polo shirt or any casual shirt looks very sharp and bold with such casual boots mentioned above. The business casual dress code is one that most default to when trying to dress the part for an event, they only need one dressier piece such as the sports jacket or the blazer that will look great with one of the casual boots aforementioned above. Besides business casual, there is smart casual and ultra-casual dress codes that are a perfect match for such casual good looking boots for men. However, there is one outfit that will never look good with boots and that is wearing shorts with boots and a blazer, that may look fashionable but I emphasized at the start of the blog that such boots are ideal for cold weather thus when the weather gets hotter, my advice is drop the boots and go for sneakers at least. By the way, I suggest men check @thursdayboots online on Instagram to see the amazing boots this company has and they even specialize in sneakers as well.

HOW TO TRANSFORM YOUR LIFE FOR THE GOOD AS A STYLISH MAN?

Transformation is a process of converting, adapting, twisting and changing a situation for the good or better. For a stylish man to be able to make systematic changes for the better in his life needs to apply these procedures and principles each and every day because it not only changes your ability to dress poorly to dress perfectly but it changes your life.

This blog will list and describe the transformations stylish men need to do for the good of their lives. So, without further ado, let's jump in.

1. Transformation will occur only if you are prepared to always dress better

This point is pretty straightforward since it emphasizes preparation. In life, you need to be prepared for the worse and there are situations that are inevitable such as death. There are people who prepare for something before diving into it. Preparation is the first step towards success because you already know what is needed, how to do it and why you are doing it. For stylish men, to be able to dress better all the time, they need to be prepared. Let's say you are having a job interview coming the following week, you want to nail the interview so badly and you really need to bag this job. Well prepare by not only studying the questions to expect and those that are needed but also dress the part. Bring on your sharp outfits like a dress shirt, a suit, a blazer and nice shoes.

Doing so is a sign that you not only care about the company by dressing properly but you are always prepared for anything and you want your first impression to be golden.

2. Transformation needs a stylish man to prioritize wearing all dress codes

Dress codes are the rules to follow in regards to dressing for that event and basically following the theme of that event. As a stylish man, in order to prioritize the types of dress codes you need to wear them so that your style transforms from good to being unstoppable. The common dress codes for men out there include: business casual, business formal, ultra casual, cocktail attire and semi-formal. All these dress codes are of paramount importance to a stylish man. These dress codes make a man to be the best dressed man in the room regardless of how expensive or inexpensive that dress code is. You can't transform your style by only sticking to one style hence there is a saying that fashion is a menu you can't keep eating the same dish.

3. Transformation needs a stylish man to invest in his education

There is a saying that a man who chooses to read has an advantage to the one who doesn't read. This is to say that education is very important and as Nelson Mandela said it "Education is the key you can use to change the world" is evident that in order for transformation to happen to your life, whatever area of your life, needs you to be knowledgeable about it. In fashion and style, there are maximum sources of information that can come to your aid. Information is a treasure and a stylish man needs to treasure reading about style like the importance of fit in style, how to dress for your body size and the habits of stylish man. The internet is filled with such information and you can easily register online for a course as well about fashion and design without actually visiting an institution. My take in terms of educating yourself about style it is to gather as much information or video content about style to be able to transform your life for the good.

4. Transformation needs a stylish man to be open to new environments and explore other styles

Change can be uncomfortable but it is a necessity and this means as stylish man, you need to let loose and be open to other environments that will boost your style such as attending fashion shows. Fashion shows are an excellent environment for seeing other people with the same interests as you and you can find yourself mingling with other stylish men, admiring each other's styles and even build good friendships with those men. Doing so ensures that you are willing to transform your style and explore other styles like trends in order to enjoy being a stylish man. I have attended a number of fashion shows since I became a stylish man and I have enjoyed the interaction there it is much soothing than sitting at home wearing clothes that only you can see.

5. Networking with other stylists can be major transformation for a stylish man

For the record, there are male stylists and these are men who deal with costumes and styling them like water flowing downhill. As a stylish man with a burning desire to transform, you need to communicate with stylists and these days of instant communication via social media and internet marketing, it really is easy to connect with a stylist (Even professional ones) who will be more than happy with help you change your style from being poorly dressed to being the best dressed man.

HOW TO WEAR A WHITE TURTLENECK FORMALLY AS A STYLISH MAN?

Turtlenecks date back to the 15th century and were usually worn by knights who would wear this classic jersey which protected their necks from the chainmail or the chainsaw. Fast forward to 2023 and turtlenecks are still worn by not the knights anymore but even fashionable and classic men. Now the question lies then, how do you wear a white turtleneck formally as a stylish man? The solutions to that question are explained in this blog post below.

1. Formal suits are to be worn with a white turtleneck

One way to wear a white turtleneck formally it is to just bring in a formal suit. This is a suit that is formal by design and the current ones we have in stores are suits with double vents and double breasted suits. Findings on the internet give many synonyms to the word "Formal", they call it evening dress, dress clothes, white tie, black tie and full evening dress. Why the color white on a turtleneck? Well because this color is the most formal and looks very clean as it slims up the silhouette of the suit thus a white turtleneck is ideal. Sources from google explain that in the late 1800s the Victorian era and till the 1900s, England was the only country to dominate American menswear and for good reason. Most people who see others wearing suits have this perception that they are like the English Men who are highly educated. Yes in theory that is proven to be a fact but a suit does not mean you are from England but it does carry with it the convenience that this man knows English and can be in charge of a business.

For the suits, as I usually write in my previous blog post, a suit needs to be well tailored or it must fit your body so that it looks good on you and colors such as navy blue, charcoal grey, black, dark green and brown are ideal for formal wear. Believe me when I say you will never go wrong with pairing a white turtleneck with these suits colors and just leave the dress shirt and ties at home.

2. White turtlenecks need to be tucked thus a belt is mandatory

That's right, a belts creates a slimmed up appearance especially if you are a thin guy. For the bigger guys with bellies, probably a belt won't work for their figure but I think suspenders are fine for that type of man because you can tuck in the turtleneck like a dress shirt and just fasten the clips if you are wearing a clip on suspender. Tucking in the turtleneck is done to project a formal look which needs you to dress up.

3. If suits are not your thing bring on an overcoat

I know there are some gents out there who don't wear suits on a daily basis like myself or don't like suits at all, there is nothing wrong with that. I think an overcoat will assist in this scenario, coats like these are super affordable even the second hands ones. A black or brown overcoat matches perfectly with a white turtleneck and nice boots or dress shoes. What I don't think will match with the coat and turtleneck is jeans because the subject of this blog post it is formal menswear.

4. It is important that you buy quality fabrics like cashmere because they can be layered with other formal pieces in your closet

This is another reason why a man needs to buy the right turtleneck not just the color white but also consider the fabric of the turtleneck. I suggest a cashmere fabric because it has a soft drape that makes it super comfortable on the skin and they provide extra warmth.

I believe a white, brown and blue turtleneck is ideal but for the purposes of this blog post, white is the preferred color since it works in bringing the formality of the outfit. This cashmere fabric on a turtleneck can also be matched with a sports jacket or blazer that is not from the suit, a leather jacket or suede jacket also works well with this turtleneck if you want to go for at least a smart casual or business casual outfit.

5. White and black are great combinations thus for footwear black boots are ideal

If you want to add combinations don't be afraid to add a black boot to the mix because you will look presentable and sharply dressed. The boot adds style too.

IMPROVEMENTS MEN WILL EXPERIENCE BY CONSTANTLY PUTTING ON SUITS

Suits are classy, elegant and a stylish addition in any man's wardrobe. Men have been wearing suits since the 1800s and research proves that the single breasted suit is the one I usually wear and my personal favorite has been around since the 1920s compared to the double breasted suit that was introduced years later and it was an attire reserved for the conservative gentleman. Research also proves that the terms suit was derived from the French word "Suivre" which means to follow and it is true, a suit must follow other parts of the outfit like the pants and shoes thus a suit refers to a jacket and trouser made from the same fabric and they need to follow each other.

This blog will state the improvements men will experience by constantly wearing suits.

1. **Suits build up your confidence**

   According to Hive & Colony, https://www.hiveandcolony.com/news/reasons-why-you-should-wear-a-suit, wearing a suit let us say the lounge suit which was first manufactured and worn in 1860 gives a man high levels of confidence and when the confidence soars, the man has a high chance for success and as long as

the suit is comfortable and the fit is nailed success
is around the corner for the man who wears a suit.

2. **Suits are a timeless outfit**

That's right, suits in nature are elegant and timeless
meaning they stand the test of time. A well fitted
three piece suit, double breasted suit, lounge suit,
frock coat and evening dress will always look classy
in 2023 and you don't have to worry about it going
out of style even in the next 20 years, suits will
definitely be king. On the other hand, fashionable
suits are trendy and trends come and go so know
the difference between classic suits and fashionable
suits.

3. **Suits are a comfortable attire**

I know there are some men who don't like wearing
suits, maybe it is because they don't love the style
or there are not into class. Whatever the reason is,
suits are one of the most comfortable attires a man
can wear, the thing that scares most men is that they
think suits are uncomfortable and too expensive for
my liking, those in my view are just theories. Suits
are very comfy and they make you look important
and give you a sense of dignity.

4. **Suits reserve respect**

   Yes this is the most important factor in suits and that is they grant a man the respect he deserves. According to Hive & Colony, every man deserves respect and wants to receive it, so why not meet respect along the way by wearing that suit of yours when going to church, to dates, to work, when travelling and to formal events such as conferences, awards, galas and other key events you have lined up to attend. I have received respect a thousand of times every time I put on my Navy Blue suit and I just love it, so can you!

5. **Suits allows you to style according to your preferences**

   Obviously there are men who want to style a suit in their own way and that is fine. Suits can be dressed down to a casual notch and there are an array of options for that, for example, when attending an informal event such as a cultural event like the Reed Dance, you can opt for the suit blazer only which you can wear casually with fitted jeans, for the shirt, I would say wear a shirt without a necktie since you are not going to the office but on its own or switch it for a t-shirt in plain colors it will do wonders for that business casual style. This option of playing with your preferences is to allow men to not be afraid to wear their own selective outfits they normally default to hence I mentioned the need of wearing a t-shirt (most men have t-shirts and wear them all the time even as an undergarment)

FAMOUS CELEBRITIES AND ACTORS WHO LOOK SHARP IN SUITS

Wearing a suit leads to a man being highly confident and when that confidence rises, his chances of success escalate drastically. Men in suits look like success and here are the popular actors and celebrities worldwide who love wearing suits which can influence any man to invest in one.

1. **Gabriel Macht (Plays Harvey Specter in legal drama show "Suits")**

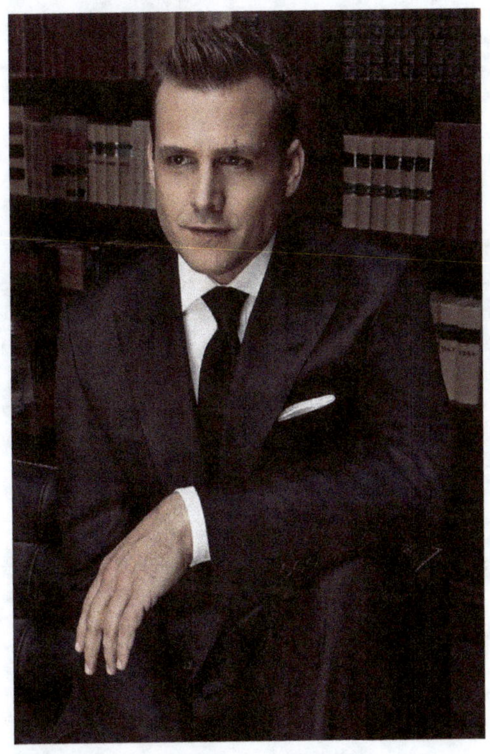

2. Jason Statham (An actor well known for his actionable stunts and in the popular movie "FAST AND FURIOUS HOBBS AND SHAW")

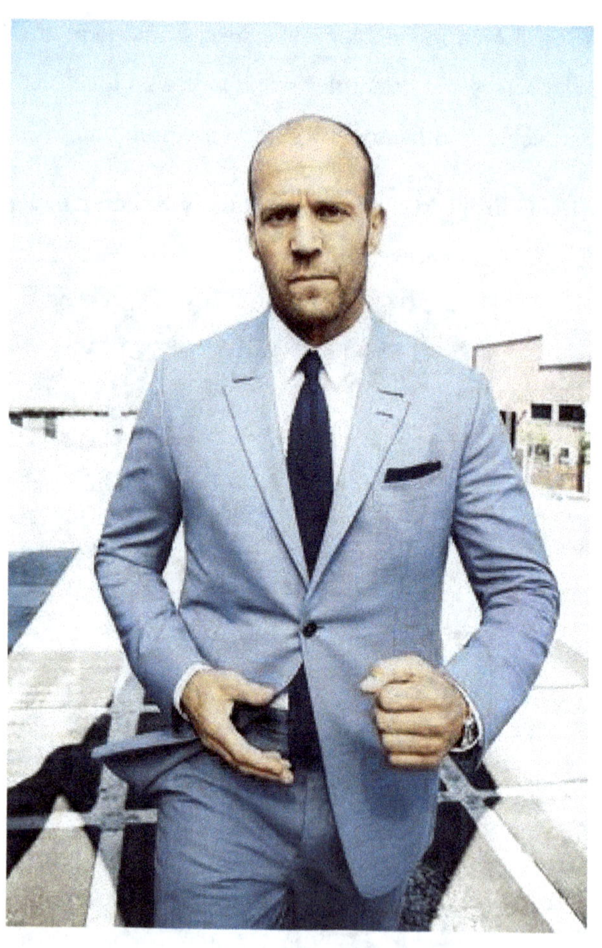

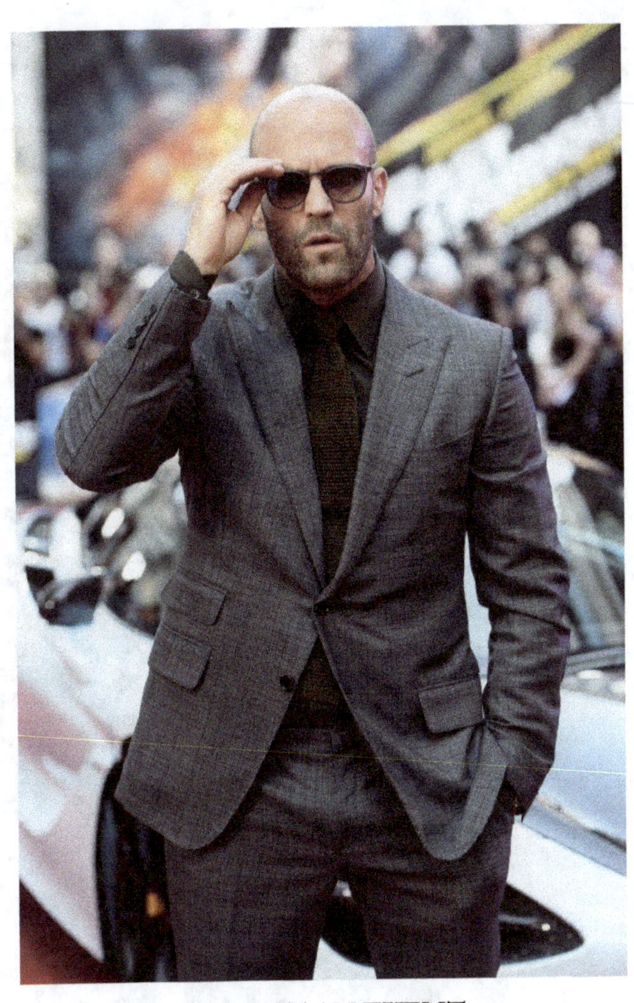

JASON STATHAM AT AN EVENT

3. Will Smith (An Actor well known in movies like "Men in black" and others)

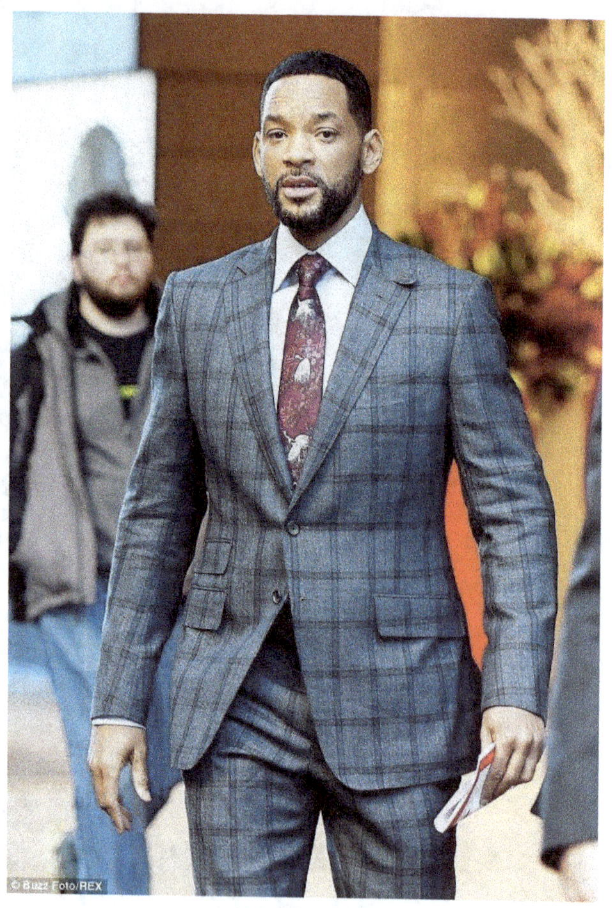

4. Tom Ellis (A prolific Actor well known as Lucifer in the supernatural series "LUCIFER" and also played the role of Will Rush in TV drama series "RUSH" that aired in 2014)

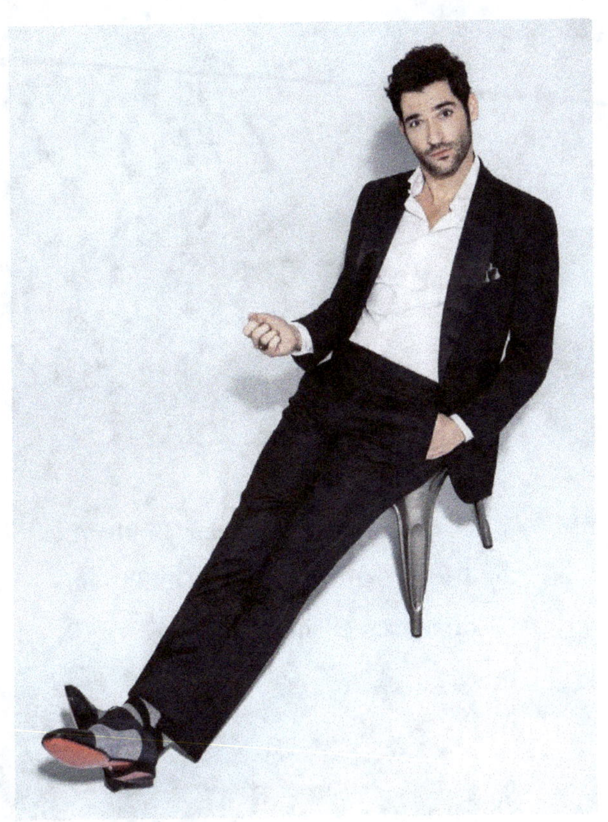

5. Chadwick Boseman (The late Wakanda actor who was known during the 2018 movie "WAKANDA")

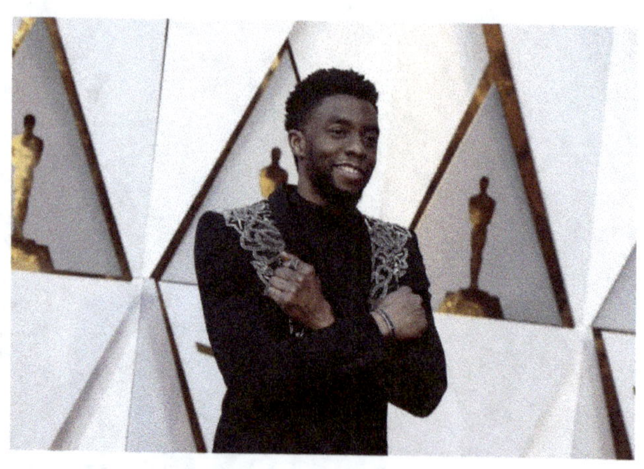

6. Damian Lewis (Played as Bobby Axelrod in TV drama show **"BILLIONS"** on showtime broadcast channel)

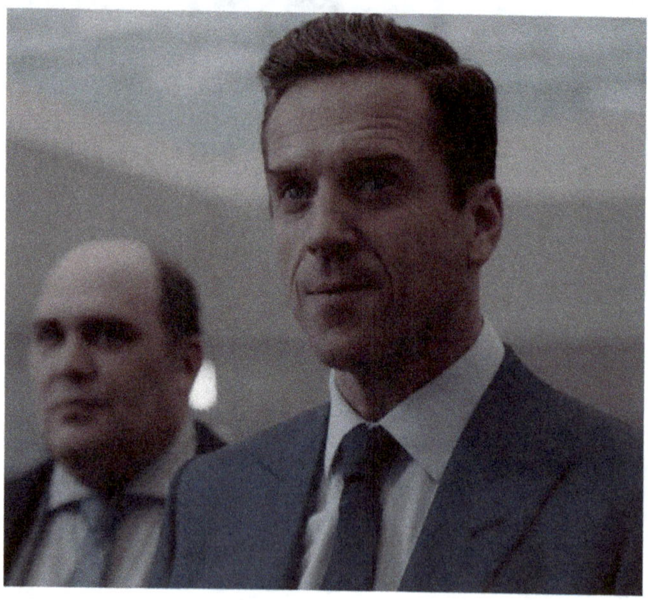

7. Grant Gustin (Played as Barry Allen AKA "THE FLASH" on CW super fictional series "FLASH")

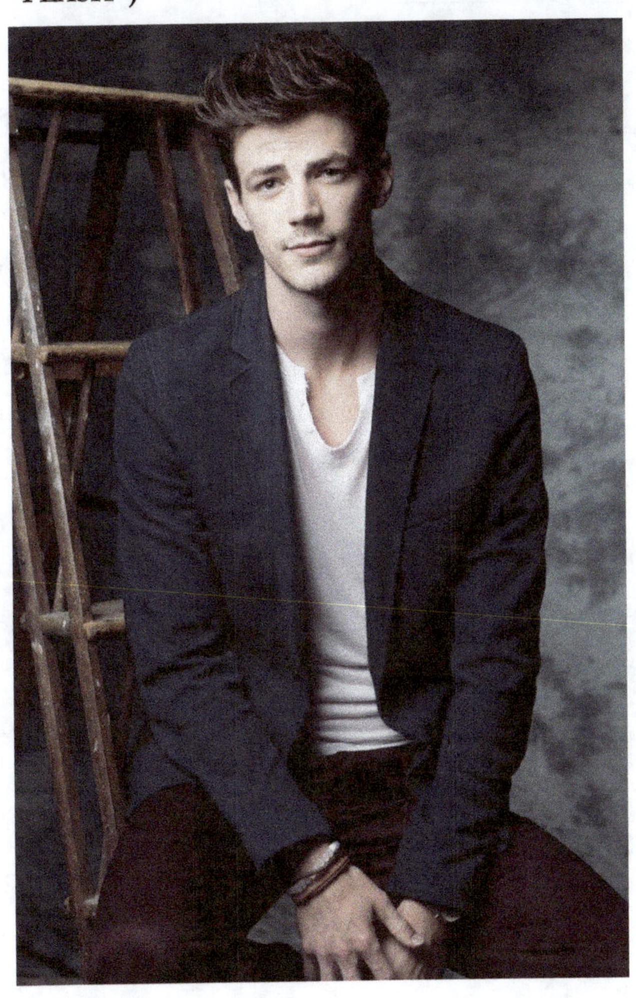

MEN WITH THE TENDENCY TO WEAR CASUAL MODE NEED HELP DRESSING ELEGANTLY

It is a fact that on God's green earth there are a bunch of men who default and usually grab casual wear outfits each and every day such as t-shirts, jeans, sneakers, sunglasses and necklaces. Whilst there is nothing wrong with attaching yourself with those clothing items, when it comes to dressing elegantly which means dressing classy, grandeur, gentility and to even charm people you need to drop those casual items like a hot potato because they don't do you any good in dressing you up a bit especially if you are to show your face to an important event. This blog will give out examples of elegant outfits' men with the tendency to wear casual wear need to start wearing to appear well dressed in the room.

Here are the 8 items men who lack in elegance need:

1. **A well fitted suit**

Okay I have to say whenever I hear the word "Suits" I get excited and for one obvious reason, a well fitted suit actually makes a man look sharp, dapper, of high status and he appears to be the well- dressed guy. Here is the benefit of wearing a fitted suit, it will last you a lifetime because suits are classic in design and they are timeless hence they will always look good even in 2023. To be a classic man, you need at least one suit in your wardrobe and I recommend men throw their eyes on these colors for their suits: Navy Blue, Grey, Brown, Burgundy, White, Dark Green and Black.

2. Have a watch to not only be on time but to accessorize elegantly in style

I have been preaching the need of men having watches since I started this blog and it is true. A watch is advantageous in that it ensures that you come to work on time and it keeps you afloat in terms of deadlines and priorities that need to be done on time. Also, a watch give you the relationship between you and style, men even those on a budget can get an affordable watch that they can wear with a suit and even with their usual casual outfits.

3. Play around with colors

The reason I am passionate about fashion and style it is because I don't back down when it comes to colors. I use colors and even in elegant style such as wearing a black tie or black tie dress code, I do ensure I throw in that bright color such as a yellow pocket square or tie. Trust me, a color will aid you to look better than the next gent in the room.

4. Wear jeans often

According to the Men's Wear Advice Blog which you can visit using this link- https://www.cliffroseforclothes.com/the-mens-wear-advice-blog , Jeans are a lifesaver in terms of needing a casual trouser you can even wear with a grandeur blazer or sports jacket. I have also pulled off a classy look with my blue denim jeans, blazer, crew neck sweater and boots. Trust me, this combo makes you look great and elegant even if you want to dress down.

5. Look after your physical appearance

This is what we call applying grooming tips to ensure your physical look appears great in the eyes of others. A shave, hair product, perfume or fragrances are all crucial elements of looking good and I suggest men try them.

6. Get amazing underwear

Yes you heard me, quality underwear such as these brands like Calvin klein are a must have and I know no one will know what underwear you stripped on but you need one for yourself.

7. Get good shoes

Not so long ago, I published a blog about shoes and the types of shoes every stylish man needs, do head over to my blog and check older posts titled "5 MISCELLANEOUS SHOES TO FALL IN LOVE WITH EVERY STYLISH MEN NEEDS IN 2023" and you will comprehend why I say get good shoes.

8. Accessorize with authority

This means practice wearing less accessories and in elegance less is more, an outfit that is too flashy becomes boring thus authority in other words control needs to be adhered to here.

MEN'S MUST HAVE PIECES THAT ARE A BOMB

Okay let me just say for the record, an outfit can be anything you put on your body and it is of no importance whether it is a designer outfit or not. However, if you want to be a stylish man with elegance and class you need to purchase and practice wearing pieces like baseball caps, chino pants, sneakers, floral shirts and white t-shirts. Why? Because such pieces are versatile and a must have in your wardrobe.

Baseball caps

Baseball caps or basketball caps as they are usually known are worn by men not only when going to watch sports like the above mentioned but they can even wear such caps when going out to meet with friends or family. Caps like these are a must have because they just hype up your street style in a major way. The trendiest style for 2023 is going to be streetwear chic so such caps are a must have if you want to be in trend this year. This cap can even be worn with a blazer layered with a hoodie or graphic t-shirt to give the style a bomb in terms of appearance. Lastly, caps like these can be worn with jeans, shorts, flip flops, sneakers and other casual ensembles you might have hence it is super versatile.

Chino pants

Pants like these are very versatile given that you can wear them casually and even dressed up. Brown chino pants for example can be worn with floral shirts, sports jackets, white dress shirt, black turtlenecks or crew neck sweaters and some nice shoes like boots even which are my favorite footwear.

Sneakers

Sneakers of course are a must have because these shoes make it easy for you to walk without having itching problems or having difficulty walking because the shoe shape is irregular. White and black sneakers in my own view are needed and they do produce a bomb of an outfit since you dress them up or dress them down.

Floral shirts

Okay, floral shirts are actually casual in nature because of the patters and prints they are made from. Shirts like these can be versatile since you can dress them up with a solid suit such as blue or grey and even dress them down with jeans or chinos and nice sneakers.

White t-shirts

Last of the items that are needed it is white t-shirts because you can dress them up and even down so they are super versatile and stylish. Such shirts are ideal since you can wear them as an undergarment or with a suit or with shorts or with jeans and will match almost any shoe you have. Thus, I urge men to wear a white t-shirt or better yet own at least 2 pairs of them.

SIMPLICITY IS THE ULTIMATE SOPHISTICATION IN CLASSIC MENSWEAR

Men who want to delve into classic menswear need to follow some guidelines in order for their classic style to stand out, to be elegant and to be timeless. Famous actor Don Draper once said in his quote "Make it simple yet significant" which means he was describing the essence of simplicity that it makes a man look classic, sharp and elegant. Take for instance the white dress shirt and white turtleneck, both are ideal for classic wear and they can be worn with suits, jeans, sports jacket and long overcoats. This blog will describe the significance of classic apparel for men and what classic style should look like.

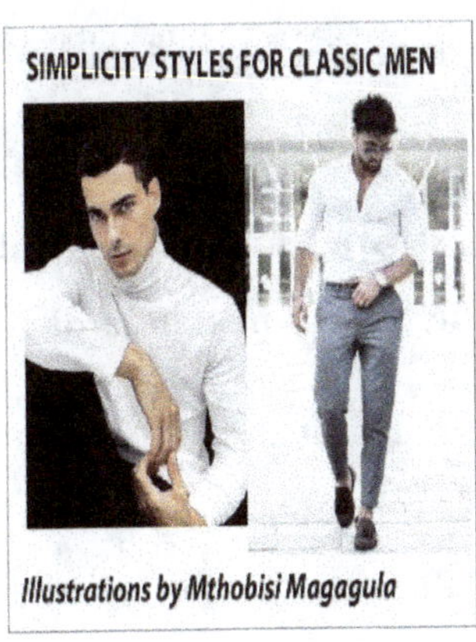

Illustrations by Mthobisi Magagula

Classic style always stands the test of time

If you can take time to research what men in the 80s or 90s wore, you will get to figure out that most wore vintage and classic apparel such as the evening dress, frock coats, flap caps for headwear and boots or black formal shoes which were worn by those men who worked in corporations and offices. In nowadays, the office environment has changed in terms of what men need to wear their best at work, now even those situated in offices no longer wear 3 piece suits but they wear their jeans, jackets and sneakers, the only time they will be seen wearing classic pieces such as the suit, blazers and formal shoes is when they have a meeting with the company staff, with clients or they are going to close a deal with investors. It's 2023 and classic style is still strong as it will never fade, even a man who can pull of a tweed suit (which we don't see these days) will still look classic, elegant and simple.

Classic style accessories such as suspenders and tie bar give your simplicity elegant standards

Okay let us not forget the accessories that certainly prove that classic style is the best style men can invest in. Accessories like these are just of high standard and they make a man look dapper and some might say he is a dandy. I have both these accessories, that is, the suspenders and tie bar and trust me they make me look high status, like I am wealthy and that is what classic accessories do to your style, they add details, make you look rich and they are to be kept simple by wearing a few at least 3 of them. The suits of today lack such classic accessories and having a tie bar and suspenders does wonders as the suspenders bring in the 90s vibe instead of the usual belts men wear and the tie bar ensures your tie doesn't drift off or blow away when the temperature gets windy all of a sudden.

Classic style is for men who prefer to look mature and not those into fashion trends as those go in and out of fashion

Classic style is my favorite style as a man into simplicity and it works for my body. I know that there are other men who don't love suits, vintage and classic apparel and that is fine, we all have our own styles. For the man who isn't into class but likes trends that are in fashion well go for it, the trendiest styles we see now are vintage t-shirts, street wear smart and we see casual shirts & tie. The thing about these trends is that they come and go thus if you don't have enough money you won't last because some are very hefty in pricing. On the other side, classic menswear will never fade and the advantage of this style is that it makes you look older or matured and that can be a good thing if you want to be taken seriously and respected.

WHY DRESSING PROPER MAKES A MAN STILLER AND MORE PRODUCTIVE?

Dressing proper as a man is a good thing and it is one of the signs of being productive. Proper in itself is a word that means still and intact and it directs you to doing something that is orderly and noble. There are many benefits of dressing proper which leads to a man being more still and productive in his life.

Credibility

This is one major reason why dressing proper is a must as a man. Credibility goes along with your reputation. If you start dressing sharp and proper as a man whether you are attending important functions or not is the first step towards productivity. The environment you work in or where you stay needs you to dress proper so that people get to entrust your reputation. Whether you are a banker, farmer, blogger, musician, lawyer, doctor or any occupation that you practice needs a man to dress pertinent for his own credibility. To be credible and for people to credit you requires a man to invest in looking his best. It can be a fitted suit, blazer, sports jacket or any proper garment a man owns goes a long way in ticking the boxes of credibility that can lead to a promotion at your workplace because your dress code is exemplary.

Credibility is a factor that leads to stillness and productivity hence men shouldn't undermine their habit of looking proper.

Great first impressions

Ryan Holiday in his book titled "Stillness is the key" talks about stillness as the key to everything. Being still means you think clearly, to making tough decisions, to maintaining high pressure environments, to making good habits, to maintaining healthy relationships , to physical excellence and experiencing moments of joy and laughter as well as being more productive.

With that being said, dressing proper firsthand is a great way to constructing first impressions and ensuring that people believe in you and more key welcoming you especially if you are job hunting. Potential employers will be convinced first that you are the right candidate for the job die to your appearance. Seeing a man with a suit and tie is already a win for that employer and you as a man have already one foot at the door to success and attaining full time employment.

Decision making

Stillness focuses on three domain parts being the mind, body and soul. A man who doesn't dress proper and is drunk when going to work or even after hours cannot make good decisions instead make poor decisions as a result of recklessness and an untidy outfit.

In the workplace, we have strategic levels and operational levels as well as an organizational structure such as who is at the top, bottom and the middle and all of these structures have people who work tirelessly to ensure the business succeeds but the main person who holds the swimming or sinking of the company is the person at the top, the CEO as some would say. That is why some CEOs when it comes to decision making don't engage in substances such as drinking because that could hurt the company's vision and mission. A leader in other words must conduct himself in a way that deems fit for professional business practices and also dress proper. A leader who is still and dresses proper is able to master and make those difficult choices because the mind, body and soul is quiet, open to suggestions, calm and more focused to make radical changes that will transform the company and push it forward ahead of its competitors. Therefore, a man who is still and dresses proper excels at decision making than a man who panics and dresses poorly.

Dressing proper communicates that you take your work seriously

Logically, a man in a suit is seen as serious, keen and focused at his own work. Dressing proper shows and it communicates a pattern that you want to go from being nothing to being something. If you are working, dressing proper shows that you are a professional committed to his duties and even if you are not working, dressing proper still communicates messages that you are a man who wants to complete tasks and on time. Imagine being invited to an event oversees, you would of course want to pick a dress code that communicates respect and seriousness.

A REVIEW OF 80s CASUAL WEAR ITEMS FOR MEN STILL RELEVANT IN 2023

The 80s fashion is predominantly one of the most key era in the fashion world. Why is that you may ask? Well it is because that was the time where we first spot the trends, styles and fashion pieces men and women wore. The common items for casual wear in the 80s was cuffed jeans, bomber jackets, cardigans, plain t-shirts, loafers, leather jackets, denim and even vintage sports jerseys. Now, fast forward to this current era of 2023, still if you take a view again (hence the review) you will see that some of these items are still worn by men and they still look good.

This blog post will list and explain the common casual items of the 80s including their history and ways to wear them even in the relevant year 0f 2023.

Bomber jackets

According to fashion beans website – https://www.fashionbeans.com/article/how-to-dress-80s/ , bomber jackets are one of the casual items for men. Style wise, bomber jackets are a great casual jacket to own and in my personal opinion they look good with fitted jeans and a nice pair of boots. To style a bomber jacket casually, a man must have denim, a t-shirt (when the weather gets hot), cap for headwear and nice sneakers with no graphics or even branded sneakers such as Puma. Okay, the example I just gave is how you can bring in a bomber jacket when the temperature gets mild to warm but you still want to wear a jacket. If the tables changed and say the weather gets cold, I believe a bomber jacket can look good with a plain turtleneck in black, white, grey, brown and blue, add jeans, add your boots and add a beanie on your head and you will sure look good under those freezing temperatures.

THE COMPULSORY BENEFITS OF BEING A WELL-DRESSED MAN

Compulsory means importance or significance. To dress in a compulsory manner needs a man to evaluate his wardrobe, look at what he regularly wears, how does he style clothes and most importantly, grooming tactics must be utilized so that he dressed properly without looking like a slob. In academics, teachers who set scripts usually mark the section "COMPULSORY" for students to see that that section must be answered before proceeding to the other assessments. In terms of men's clothing, there are compulsory benefits of always looking the part and this blog post will list and explain the convenience of being a well-dressed (without wearing a three piece suit)

1. **Being well dressed grants you the respect you deserve**

Charles Hix once said "Looking good isn't self-importance, it is self-respect". This entirely means that when you dress well, you are showing the world that you respect yourself and with that respect comes solitude, acceptance and assertiveness. Truly, I have seen this happen to me, when I look great even in my casual such as styling boots with jeans and a sports jacket, I get the acceptance from people and they treat you like you are high status.

2.   Being well dressed shows self-confidence

A person who adopts self-confidence is one that has high levels of self-esteem, is fully aware of what's going on and is flexible in every obstacle that is standing in the way. Okay, there are many confident people in the world but before you actually spot them based on what they say, do and act, first the eyes will see the dress code and from there they will make a conclusion of whether this person is confident or shy. A man wearing a leather jacket is seen as very confident because those who wear leather jackets are actually a bad ass or so it seems.

3.   Being well dressed signals maturity

It is a fact that teenagers for example are seen as teens because of their juvenile way of dressing. Whereas, a man whether young or old wearing a well fitted blazer or a suit depending on your financial availability is seen as mature, sane, capable of making sound decisions and behaves like a gentleman.

4.   Being well dressed signals success

I have been reading this book titled "Design your life" by Cornelia Shipley and as I was perusing chapter 4 which was dubbed "Winning the game, define success for yourself" and this book has made me to think long and hard about success, on the surface we all want success and some even go to extra lengths to acquire it. In this book, the author has a series of questions lined up for the readers such as "What would make you to have joy and real meaning in your life? What do you see yourself becoming? What would bring joy to your work? And so forth.

In terms of style, I truly believe a stylish man or any man can be successful by dressing the part, applying Charles Hix's quote and learn more as well as practice being that man who can dress for success. You don't need to have gazillions of money to be a stylish man or buy the latest fancy brands but you need to understand your style, what you prefer and what colors suit your complexion. By the way, I have a previously published blog post about success titled "Grand outfits are magnets of success" which will also give you a clear picture of how to use style to your advantage.

5. **Being well dressed shows that you gradually taking your life seriously**

Okay, there comes a point in life whereby a man has to face the music and take his life seriously, it may be a life event that can cause it such as illness, loss of a family member, the age factor, changes in environment or life itself taking a negative spin. All these events are guaranteed to shake a man's mindset to take serious changes, the author Cornelia in the book "Design your life", the writer points out that each day is an opportunity to implement your plan, be it you want to start a business, avoid childish acts, prioritizing family time, investing in meaningful friendships, saving for rainy days and other essential plans. On top of that, in my style opinion, to show the people you see daily that you are serious about your life, dress the part and look like the man in charge of your life.

WHY MEN NEED TO HAVE BLACK T-SHIRTS FOUR SEASONS IN A YEAR?

Black is a classy color and it is one of the most worn colors out there in the world. Having a black item in your possession is adequate for your style needs and it is the most versatile color you can ever wear. Black has numerous advantages such as it can hide stains and dirt but the major advantages of having black especially on t-shirts is that it helps men to dress better. This blog post will disseminate the reasons why men need to have a black t-shirt at their disposal each year throughout the four seasons.

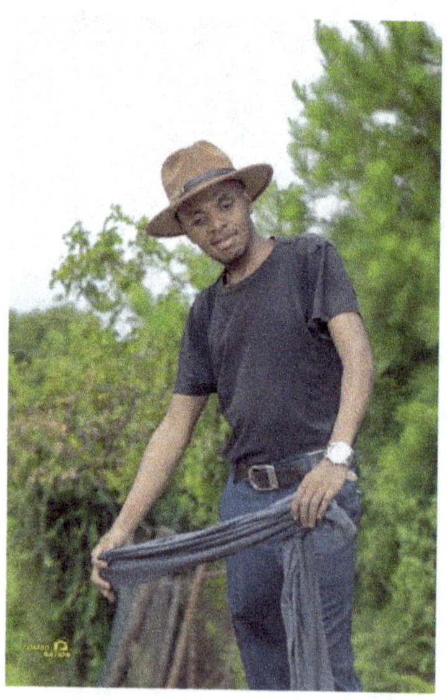

1.   Black is versatile an all fronts

One major reason why wearing all black or a black t-shirt to be specific is that it is super versatile since you can wear it on all occasions and events plus it works well with other pieces in your wardrobe. Imagine you have one suit, one trouser, one boot, one watch, one or two accessories and you need to have a t-shirt, black is the obvious choice since you can dress it up with that one suit and even dress it down casually with that jean and boot. Also, versatility goes hand in hand with being practical thus having a black item especially a t-shirt is needed for your outfit to look attractive and credible.

2.   Black is refined and ideal for formal wear

Whether it is winter, spring, summer or autumn, all of these four seasons cannot ruin the color black because it is ideal for all seasons and for formal wear it ticks all the boxes. According to https://gentlemangazette.com, men wear black because they believe it will add formality to their outfit and I agree. Black is ideal for formal style and when in doubt wear that color if you need to look great and on point. Also, if it makes you feel better, popular actors such as Idris Elba have worn black both on and off screen so can you man!

3.   Black is modern

Black is just futuristic and primal because it is one of those colors that will always look modern, sleek and fashionable too. A black suit is one example of modern menswear and although the silhouette of black suits are no longer the same as black tie, the color still is appealing and the most worn by even women.

4. Black is vintage

According to the Gentleman's Gazette, https://gentlemangazette.com, in the 60 to 70s men worn this color and it is color used for black movement and those historical events Shirts such as long sleeve shirts and polos were worn widely by men of all ages hence black is a vintage color that never fades no matter what the occasion is. Black is also a respectful color and for a man who wants to look like a gentleman, black is the color to go for since it is vintage, timeless and elegant plus it will slim up your appearance.

5. Black t-shirts can be used as an undergarment

Except for summer and spring where the weather is usually favorable and sunny, black t-shirts can be used as a starting piece or an undergarment when planning to layer them with sports jackets, suits, overcoats, flannel shirts and sweaters when the season is about to be winter. This is super practical and easy to execute because a black t-shirt paired with a suit actually ensures you feel warm instead of wearing the black t-shirt on its own. It is not only white t-shirts or vests that can be an undergarment, even black t-shirts can function in the exact same way.

6. Black is an ideal color for dressing for work and interviews

Okay this is true and very easy to do. A black t-shirt and even a dress shirt on a cold day, hot day, spring day or windy day is perfect because it is an appropriate color for dressing for work and also for nailing the interview in style. For example, a black suit, shirt, necktie or shoes in black do dress a man to look the part and elegant. Lastly, to dress for success, snatch black pieces in your wardrobe you will make your outfit seem easier and well put together plus you will look simple yet presentable.

CLASSIC STYLES MEN NEED TO WEAR FROM THE FICTIONAL BRITISH SECRET AGENT MOVIES

Ever watched movies from the British? Well if you have you will notice a few things there, first the amazing stunts and action scenes and the costumes the actors and actresses wear. One movie that love watching and the one that also propelled me to write this blog post it is "SKYFALL" and for many reasons, this movie will keep me at the edge of my seat and most importantly, it has one of the greatest spy agent known as James Bond who is portrayed by Daniel Craig.

This blog is actually a review of the secret agent Movies and there are quite plenty that were released even in the 19th century to early 20th century such as: Our Man in Havana (released 1959), 39 Steps (1959), The Greater Good (2015) and my personal favorite, the kingsman the golden circle (2017). Also, I suggest men check out my previous blog post "Kingsman movies are a good reference for men lacking in classic style and manners" to read about such movies.

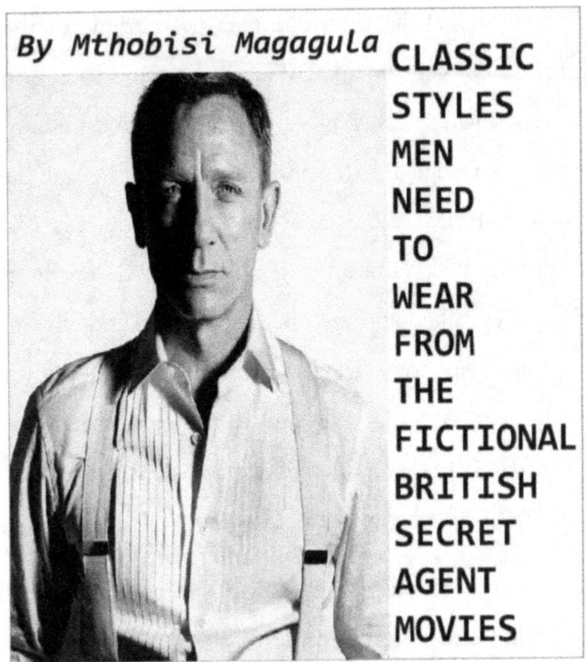

Skyfall movie reveals James Bond wearing suspenders hence men need them

Okay believe me when I say this movie is worth sacrificing your time by watching it and you will be blown away with its' content such as the scenes, visuals , bombings and most importantly if you are a man who loves classic style, the costumes and outfits are very exquisite. This movie was made by Sony and produced by Paramount pictures production with actors and actresses playing their part in making this movie watchable. The thing with these secret agents is that they have an international intrigue to them since the spy travels outside Britain or England to fight the bad guys elsewhere. This movie has James Bond known as 007 which is his stage name and this name is the one he is known for business and even the bad guys know this. Okay in terms of style, James Bond wears suspenders in the movie, I have talked about suspenders before and why men need them. Suspenders are classy and elegant plus they are ideal for men with big bellies since they hold their pants upright. Also, these are a perfect replacement for belts and they add a bit of spice to your classic apparel.

Skyfall movie reveals James Bond wearing black tie dress code hence men need one

Black tie dress code is an outfit that is more formal and men wear such attires when attending prestigious events such as Weddings, Galas, Awards and fashion shows. This is an outfit that needs a white dress shirt, black suit with a shawl lapel and for the shoes to maintain the rule of formality keep them simple with black color like black oxfords or even black boots that can be dressed up. Men need black tie for when they need to attend formal events or gatherings and they make them look sharp, clean, neat and obviously classy.

Skyfall movie reveals James Bond wearing a grey suit hence men need one

Okay I have talked about grey as neutral color in my previous blog posts and I truly believe this color here is a must have because of its versatility. Grey can be dressed up or down but in this movie we see a dressed up version of the British secret agent and he goes for lighter dress shirts like white and even a grey necktie, The details in terms of accessories are very muted because classic style doesn't need so much details and colors. In the suit you will see a white presidential fold pocket square which adds a bit of flare in the classic style hence I suggest men to buy a grey suit as one of their first suit colors, then buy navy blue, brown, red and black.

List of latest spy and secret agents shows on Netflix men need to watch:

Besides Skyfall, below are other movies with their year of release men need to check out:

- The Recruits (2022)
- In from the cold (2022)
- Kleo (2022)
- Spycraft (2021)
- Caliphate (2020)

- The spy 2019)

- Traitors (2019)

- Pine Gap (2018)

Visit https://www.netflix.com>browse>genre for more information

THANK YOU

Dear Readers,

As I pen down these final words, my heart swells with gratitude. Thank you for allowing me the privilege of being a small part of your journey. Remember, fashion isn't just about what you wear, but how you wear it. May you stride confidently, embrace your uniqueness, and let your style be a testament to the extraordinary person you are. Here's to a future where every outfit tells a story and every step forward is a declaration of self-love.

With sincere thanks,

Mthobisi Magagula

Special Gift

For every review we receive, each individual will be rewarded with a e-certificate signed by Mthobisi Magagula and a specially crafted personal note by us.

Write your review on any of the platforms where our book is listed. Do mention your name and city there for verification.

DM or TAG US at any social media platforms, and avail the benefits.

Our Social Media All In One Link: bento.me/geniuswords